KT-498-544

Medical Microbiology
made memorable

Steven H. Myint MD MRCP DipClinMicro
Professor of Clinical Microbiology, University of Leicester Medical School, Leicester, UK

Simon Kilvington PhD
Clinical Scientist, Public Health Laboratory, Leicester, UK

Anthony Maggs MB PhD MRCPath
Clinical Lecturer, University of Leicester Medical School, Leicester, UK

R. Andrew Swann MA BM BCh FRCPath
Consultant Microbiologist, Leicester Royal Infirmary, Leicester, UK

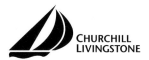

CHURCHILL LIVINGSTONE

EDINBURGH LONDON NEW YORK PHILADELPHIA SYDNEY TORONTO 1999

CHURCHILL LIVINGSTONE
An imprint of Harcourt Brace and Company Limited

© Harcourt Brace & Company Limited 1999

⊅ is a registered trade mark of Harcourt Brace and
Company Limited

The right of Professor S. H. Myint, Dr S. Kilvington,
Dr A. Maggs, and Dr R. A. Swann to be identified as
authors of this work has been asserted by them in
accordance with the Copyright, Designs and Patents
Act 1988.

All rights reserved. No part of this publication may be
reproduced, stored in a retrieval system, or transmitted
in any form or by any means, electronic, mechanical,
photocopying, recording or otherwise, without either
the prior permission of the publishers (Churchill
Livingstone, Robert Stevenson House, 1–3 Baxter's
Place, Leith Walk, Edinburgh EH1 3AF, UK) or a licence
permitting restricted copying in the United Kingdom
issued by the Copyright Licensing Agency Ltd,
90 Tottenham Court Road, London, W1P 0LP UK.

First published 1999

ISBN 0 443 06135 1

British Library Cataloguing in Publication Data
A catalogue record for this book is available from the
British Library.

Library of Congress Cataloging in Publication Data
A catalog record for this book is available from the
Library of Congress.

Medical knowledge is constantly changing. As new
information becomes available, changes in treatment,
procedures, equipment and the use of drugs become
necessary. The authors and the publishers have,
as far as it is possible, taken care to ensure that the
information given in this text is accurate and up to date.
However, readers are strongly advised to confirm that
the information, especially with regard to drug usage,
complies with current legislation and standards of
practice.

The
publisher's
policy is to use
**paper manufactured
from sustainable forests**

Printed in China

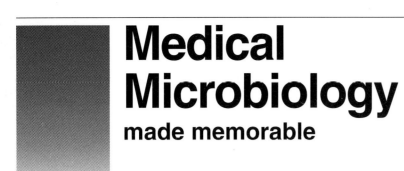

Medical
Microbiology
made memorable

For Churchill Livingstone:

Commissioning Editor: Timothy Horne
Project Editor: Janice Urquhart
Project Controller: Frances Affleck
Design Direction: Sarah Cape
Illustrator: Evi Antoniou
Page Make-up: Kate Walshaw

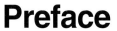

Preface

This book has principally arisen because of the changes in undergraduate medical education that mean that courses now consist of core knowledge and emphasise student-directed learning. It has also been written because biological science undergraduates have asked for a short book on medical aspects of microbiology to supplement their texts on basic microbiology. This book is aimed at both sets of students and should be used in conjunction with supplementary reading. It will not provide all the information that either student should know but forms a basis for the understanding of microbial infections.

Infections are the commonest cause of illness

Worldwide, infections cause more illness than cardiovascular disease or cancer. In developing countries they are still the most frequent reason for a patient to see his physician. This situation has not changed since the advent of antibiotics. Micro-organisms evolve faster than either man

or the pharmaceutical industry. They will always remain a threat to man's health and, possibly, survival as a species.

Infections are the commonest cause of treatable illness

Most bacterial diseases are amenable to antibiotic therapy. Although we are not there yet, the situation is also improving with diseases due to other micro-organisms. Treatment often cures infection. Most other illnesses are treated palliatively.

To be unable to understand the nature of micro-organisms, their detection and treatment would be a serious failing in any doctor. We hope that this book will ensure that does not happen.

Leicester   *S. H. M.*
1999   *S. K.*
                              A. M.
                              R. A. S.

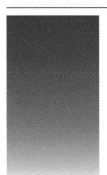

Acknowledgements

'The world is divided into people who do things — and people who get the credit'

Dwight Morrow

Much of this book has been based on many years of teaching to medical students at Leicester and elsewhere. Their input, albeit involuntary, has been invaluable. Of course we have also been, and still are, students ourselves, so to our teachers we owe a great debt.

It is our wives and families, however, to whom we owe the most gratitude as they have put up with our continuing disappearance to word processors during 'family time'.

We also wish to thank for visual material, Professor Ian Lauder, Professor Jim Lowe, Dr George Pohl and Hewlett-Packard, Mr Sudhir Sikotra, Dr Elizabeth Watkin, and Dr Kevin West. For review of the manuscript we would like to thank Lih Chyn 'Joseph' Lu.

Contents

Principles of infectious disease

1. Introduction to micro-organisms   2
2. Viruses — the basic facts   4
3. Bacteria — the basic facts   6
4. Fungi — the basic facts   8
5. Protozoa — the basic facts   10
6. Helminths — the basic facts   12
7. Viroids, prions and virinos   14

   Short answer questions 1
   Basic microbiology   16

8. Epidemiology of infectious diseases   18
9. Pathogenesis of infectious disease   20
10. Pathology of infectious disease   22
11. Innate host defences to infectious disease   24
12. Adaptive host response to infectious disease   26

   Short answer questions 2
   Immunity to infection   28

13. Diagnosis of infectious disease   30

Diseases caused by micro-organisms

14. Upper respiratory tract infections   34
15. Lower respiratory tract infections   36
16. Meningitis   38

   Case study 1   40

17. Encephalitis and other nervous system infections   42
18. Eye infections   44
19. Viral skin rashes   46
20. Cutaneous infections — bacterial and fungal   48
21. Gastrointestinal infections   50
22. Hepatitis and pancreatitis   52
23. Infections of the heart   54
24. Urinary tract infections   56
25. Genital tract infections   58

   Case study 2   60

26. Obstetric and neonatal infections   62
27. Infections of bone, joints and muscle   64
28. Septicaemia   66

   Case study 3   68

29. Acquired immunodeficiency syndrome (AIDS)   70
30. Infectious mononucleosis and other systemic infections   72

31. Infections of the immunocompromised host   74
32. Zoonoses   76

   Case study 4   78

33. Malaria   80

   Case study 5   82

34. Other tropical infections   84
35. Pyrexia of unknown origin   88
36. New and re-emerging infectious diseases   90

Control of infectious disease

37. Principles of hospital infection control   94

   Case study 6   96

38. Sterilisation and disinfection   98
39. Food, water and public health microbiology   100
40. Antibacterials — the principles   102
41. Antibacterial therapy — the practice   104

   Case study 7   106

42. Antiviral therapy   108
43. Antifungal therapy   110
44. Antiprotozoal and antihelminthic therapy   112
45. Non-drug control of infection   114
46. Genetically modified micro-organisms (GMOS) in the environment and biotechnology   115
47. Immunisation to infectious disease   116

Appendices

Appendix 1 Answers   120

Appendix 2 The language of microbiology   122

Appendix 3 Commonly used abbreviations   126

Appendix 4 Notifiable diseases (UK)   128

Appendix 5 Common helminth infections of humans   129

Appendix 6 Newly emerging pathogens and diseases   130

Appendix 7 Examples of common disinfectants and antiseptics   131

Appendix 8 Vaccines available in the UK   130

Further reading   133

Index   135

Principles of infectious disease

Introduction to micro-organisms

Micro-organisms are mostly harmless, **non-pathogenic**, and indeed may be beneficial. It is estimated that a human body has about 10^{14} cells, but only 10% of these are human in origin; the rest is almost entirely microbial flora. **Medical microbiology** is the study of microscopic organisms and their effect on man. It encompasses their biology, diagnosis, treatment and prevention.

There is a vast array of agents that are capable of causing human disease (**Table 1.1**). A 'family tree' of all living organisms is shown opposite (**Fig. 1.1**). This tree, with its three main branches, is very different from that suggested twenty years ago and has come about because of advances in molecular biology. The eukaryotic domain is a single group containing an almost unbelievable amount of diversity, from single-celled amoebae through worms, fungi and plants right up to complex animals such as humans.

The prokaryotes are divided up into two fundamentally separate domains: the Archaea and **Bacteria**. But just because many bacteria look the same under the microscope, it doesn't follow that they will behave similarly — indeed there is as much difference between the genes of the bacteria *Treponema pallidum* and *Staphylococcus aureus* as there is between those of human beings and sweet corn!

- The *Archaea* are a group of prokaryotes that live in extreme conditions such as thermal pools. Whilst they may be very important to the health of natural environments, they are not known to cause human infection.
- The *Bacteria*, however, are very significant when it comes to human health, both because some of them must live on us or in us if we are to remain healthy (our **commensal** flora)

and because some of them are capable of causing disease.
- *Eukarya*, with their larger, more diverse and complicated cells (**Fig. 1.2**), include fungi (yeasts and moulds) and parasites (single-celled protozoa and helminths).
- Viruses, viroids and prions are not truly 'living' agents, but are transmissible and able to replicate.

If we are to reduce morbidity and mortality from infection, a number of issues must be considered. The environment must be managed through public health measures to reduce the chances of contact with virulent micro-organisms. In hospitals, this process is called 'infection control' and it includes steps to ensure that patients with hazardous agents do not disseminate them to others. Innate and specific immunity are clearly important in determining the outcome of contact with pathogenic organisms; we must understand how immunity works, what happens when it is disturbed through modern medical treatments and how it might be increased by methods such as immunisation. Disease must be diagnosed quickly and accurately, either clinically or through laboratory methods, before it has spread to others or the individual is too ill to be saved. We must develop and apply high-quality, evidence-based treatments which include the prompt and appropriate use of drugs; the ideal antibiotic will kill the infecting micro-organism but not the commensal bacterial flora or the patient, and yet will not lead to antibiotic resistance amongst virulent bacteria over time. Infections are extremely common, and it is vital that all medical doctors thoroughly understand basic microbiology if they are to prevent, diagnose and treat infections effectively.

TABLE 1.1

Basic features of infectious agents

			Prokaryotes	Eukaryotes		
	Prions	Viruses/viroids	Bacteria	Protozoa	Fungi	Helminths
Living?	No	No	Yes	Yes	Yes	Yes
Self-replication	Yes/No	No	Yes	Yes	Yes	Yes
Size	Atomic microscope	Electron microscope	Microscope	Microscope	Microscope/naked eye	Microscope/naked eye
Nucleus	No	No	No	Yes	Yes	Yes
Nucleic acid	No (only protein)	DNA or RNA	DNA & RNA	DNA & RNA	DNA & RNA	DNA & RNA
Cell structure	No cell	No cell	Bacterial	Eukaryotic	Eukaryotic	Eukaryotic
Cell wall	–	–	Yes (peptidoglycan)	No	Yes (chitin)	No
Multicellular	–	–	No	No	Variable	Yes
Ribosomes	–	–	70S	80S	80S	80S
Internal organelles	–	–	No	Yes	Yes	Yes

FIG 1.1 The 'tree of life'

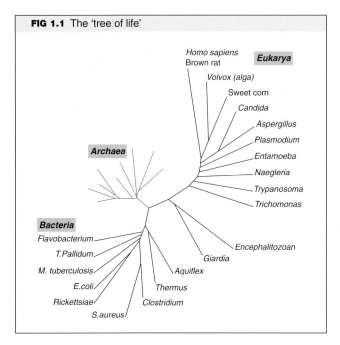

FIG 1.2 Relative sizes of infectious agents

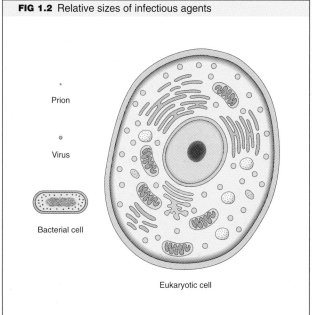

2

Viruses — the basic facts

Termed after the Latin for 'poison', viruses are the smallest and simplest of the agents of infection in man, with the possible exception of prions (**Fig. 2.1**). They are both the commonest organisms found in the environment and the most frequent cause of human infection. The following properties distinguish them from living (prokaryotic and eukaryotic) cells:

- They are acellular and have a simple organisation.
- They possess *either* **DNA** or **RNA** in the same structure.
- They cannot replicate independently of host cells.

They can exist extracellularly as **virions** with few, if any, enzymes and intracellularly when they 'hijack' the host biochemical machinery to produce copies of virion components.

Virus structure and morphology

Virions are 15–400 nm in diameter and exhibit one of five basic morphologies (**Fig. 2.2**). They basically consist of a shell, called a **capsid** which may be icosahedral or helical in shape. Capsids may be surrounded by an outer membrane, called the envelope. There is a fifth structure type, termed complex, with a capsid structure which is neither helical nor icosahedral; complex viruses may also possess an **envelope**. The capsid is an arrangement of protein subunits, termed protomers or capsomeres. Enclosed within the capsid is the genetic material, which is either RNA or DNA, and may be single stranded or double stranded. If single-stranded RNA, this may be capable of acting as messenger RNA, so-called **positive-sense**, or will have to be made into a complementary copy to do so, termed **negative-sense**. Some genomes are also segmented, such as rotaviruses.

Classification of viruses

Viruses are currently classified into different taxonomic groups on the basis of:

- the nature of the host (animal, plant, bacterial, insect or fungal)
- whether they possess an envelope
- the type of nucleic acid they possess
- the morphology of their capsid
- the diameter of the virion or nucleocapsid
- their immunological properties
- the intracellular location of viral replication
- their clinical features, i.e. disease(s) caused and method of transmission.

The first three of these are the most commonly used. In addition, there is a commonly used term 'arbovirus' which encompasses a range of virus families which are all *ar*thropod-*bo*rne. The term 'phage' is used to denote viruses which parasitise bacteria, i.e. **bacteriophage**.

The range of viruses that infect humans is shown in **Table 2.1**.

Viral replication

All viruses make copies of themselves in the intracellular phase. The major difference between viruses is their strategy for genome replication. All viruses have to generate messenger RNA to produce protein and nucleic acid copies. The route by which they do this forms the Baltimore system of classification (**Fig. 2.3**).

The end-result of viral infection may be **lysis** of the cell, **lysogeny** where the host cell is not destroyed but continues to support viral replication, or **latency** where there is little, or no, viral replication. In the latter states the viral genome may be integrated into that of the host.

Viral replication is not perfect, and mutant genomes are also made: this is the means by which viruses evolve. Non-replicative mutants are termed **defective-interfering (DI)** particles, which interfere with the replication of the initial virus.

The protean manifestations of virus infection

Viruses produce acute, persistent or chronic and latent infections. In latent infections the virus is dormant for long periods and may not produce detectable virions. Apart from the classic diseases, viruses are increasingly recognised as causes of cancer (e.g. hepatoma) and autoimmune disorders. It should also be noted that there are many 'orphan' viruses, such as adeno-associated viruses and hepatitis G virus, for which a disease has yet to be established.

TABLE 2.1

Major virus families that infect humans

Family	Nucleic acid	Envelope	Capsid	Example
Adenoviridae	dsDNA	No	Cubic	Adenovirus
Arenaviridae	ssRNA	Yes	Complex	Lassa
Bunyaviridae	ssRNA	Yes	Helical	Hantaan
Caliciviridae	ssRNA	No	Cubic	Norwalk virus
Coronaviridae	ssRNA	Yes	Helical	229E
Filoviridae	ssRNA	Yes	Helical	Marburg
Flaviviridae	ssRNA	Yes	Cubic	Hepatitis C
Hepadnaviridae	dsDNA	No	Cubic	Hepatitis B
Herpesviridae	dsDNA	Yes	Cubic	Epstein–Barr virus
Orthomyxoviridae	ssRNA	Yes	Helical	Influenza A virus
Papovaviridae	dsDNA	No	Cubic	Papillomavirus
Paramyxoviridae	ssRNA	Yes	Helical	Respiratory syncytial virus
Parvoviridae	ssDNA	No	Cubic	B19
Picomaviridae	ssRNA	No	Cubic	Rhinovirus
Poxviridae	dsDNA	Yes	Complex	Molluscum contagiosum
Reoviridae	dsRNA	No	Cubic	Rotavirus
Retroviridae	ssRNA	Yes	Complex	Human immunodeficiency virus
Rhabdoviridae	ssRNA	Yes	Helical	Rabies
Togaviridae	ssRNA	Yes	Cubic	Rubella

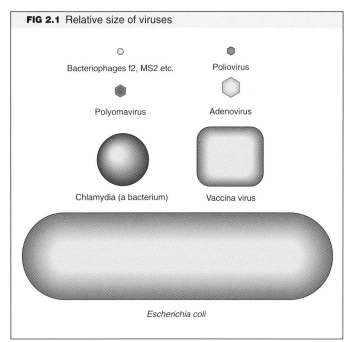

FIG 2.1 Relative size of viruses

Bacteriophages f2, MS2 etc.

Poliovirus

Polyomavirus

Adenovirus

Chlamydia (a bacterium)

Vaccina virus

Escherichia coli

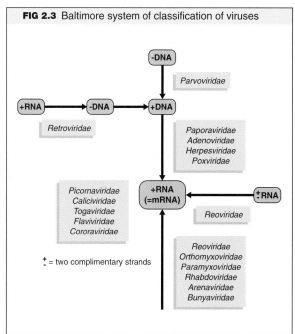

FIG 2.3 Baltimore system of classification of viruses

-DNA

Parvoviridae

+RNA → -DNA → +DNA

Retroviridae

Paporaviridae
Adenoviridae
Herpesviridae
Poxviridae

Picornaviridae
Caliciviridae
Togaviridae
Flaviviridae
Cororaviridae

+RNA (=mRNA)

±RNA

Reoviridae

$\pm$ = two complimentary strands

Reoviridae
Orthomyxoviridae
Paramyxoviridae
Rhabdoviridae
Arenaviridae
Bunyaviridae

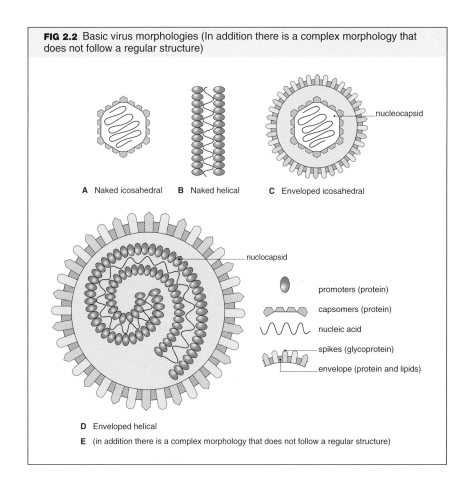

FIG 2.2 Basic virus morphologies (In addition there is a complex morphology that does not follow a regular structure)

nucleocapsid

A Naked icosahedral   **B** Naked helical   **C** Enveloped icosahedral

nuclocapsid

promoters (protein)

capsomers (protein)

nucleic acid

spikes (glycoprotein)

envelope (protein and lipids)

D Enveloped helical

E (in addition there is a complex morphology that does not follow a regular structure)

3

Bacteria — the basic facts

Bacteria are divided into two main groups by chemical staining and light microscopy: **Gram-positive** and **Gram-negative**. The Gram stain, established in the 19th century, involves fixing of the bacterium with heat or alcohol and staining with crystal violet, and then iodine. If the bacterium is Gram-positive, this blue stain is then resistant to decolorisation with alcohol or acetone. Gram-negative bacteria are decolorised and then counter-stained with a red dye, safranin or carbol-fuchsin. The differential staining is based on a major difference in the cell wall (**Fig. 3.1**). Both have a lipid bilayer **cytoplasmic membrane** with various inserted proteins, the most important of which are membrane-spanning **permeases** that control active transport of nutrients and waste products into and out of the cell. A complex web of cross-linked **peptidoglycan** outside the cytoplasmic membrane provides the cell with mechanical strength. It is particularly abundant in Gram-positives, when it also contains strands of **teichoic** and **lipoteichoic acid**. Gram-negatives have an additional **outer membrane** enclosing a thin layer of peptidoglycan and enzymes within the **periplasm**, an environment controlled by the movement of substrates through membrane **porins**. Some bacterial species may have a loosely-adherent **polysaccharide capsule** exterior to the cell wall and possibly additional structures which project from the cell surface:

- **Flagellae** are whip-like cords, typically 0.02 μm thick, 10 μm in length. A cell may have 1–20 flagellae which, when rotated, lead to the movement of the bacterial cell.
- **Fimbriae** (also called pili) are hair-like structures typically 6 nm thick, 1 μm long. There may be up to 1000 per cell, and they are composed of proteins (**adhesins**) that enable the specific attachment of the bacterium to its target.
- **Sex pili** are straighter, thicker and longer than fimbriae. A pilus can extend from one cell to another 'receptive' bacterium and allows the transfer of **plasmid DNA**.

Most bacteria that commonly affect human health are described in **Table 3.1**, although there are a few that do not take up the Gram stain:

- *Mycobacterium* species, have a thick waxy coat which can be detected by the **Ziehl–Neelsen** stain
- *Chlamydia, Rickettsia* and *Mycoplasma* species, which do not have conventional cell walls; specialised techniques are used for their visualisation and culture
- the spirochaetes (*Borrelia, Leptospira* and *Treponema*).

Bacteria may be small, but what they do, they do well. Most that cause disease grow at human body temperature (37°C). The majority grow in air (**aerobes**) but can grow without it (**facultative anaerobes**); a few can only grow in the absence of oxygen (true **anaerobes**). Bacteria multiply by **binary fission**, each cell dividing into two 'daughter' cells, and, with division times as short as 20 minutes, their growth can be explosive (**Table 3.2**). Although mutations can occur in chromosomal DNA, their rapid adaptability is due to the ability to exchange DNA:

- Some bacteria take up DNA from solution outside the cell and incorporate it into their chromosomes (**transformation**).
- Many cells contain small circular pieces of DNA, called **plasmids**, in addition to their chromosome. Plasmids may contain genes for virulence factors and antibiotic resistance, and they can move from one bacterial cell to another (**conjugation**).
- Bacterial cells can be infected by specialised viruses, called **bacteriophages** or **phages**, which move between cells, sometimes carrying genes for virulence factors (**transduction**).

The great majority of bacteria do not cause disease and live quite happily, and often to our benefit, on us or in us as **commensals** (**Fig. 3.2**). However, under some conditions, these, or more virulent micro-organisms, cause infections which may be life-threatening.

TABLE 3.1	
Gram stain reactions of common bacteria	
Gram-positive	**Gram-negative**
Cocci (= round)	
Staphylococcus (clusters)	*Neisseria* (pairs)
Streptococcus (chains/pairs)	*Moraxella*
Enterococcus (chains)	
Bacilli (= rod-like)	
Listeria	*Enterobacteriaceae*
Bacillus	● *Escherichia*
Corynebacterium	● *Klebsiella*
	● *Salmonella*
	● *Shigella*
	● *Proteus*
	Pseudomonas
	Haemophilus
	Bordetella
	Legionella
	Campylobacter
	Helicobacter
	Vibrio
Clostridium (anaerobic)	*Bacteroides* (anerobic)

FIG 3.1 The bacterial cell wall

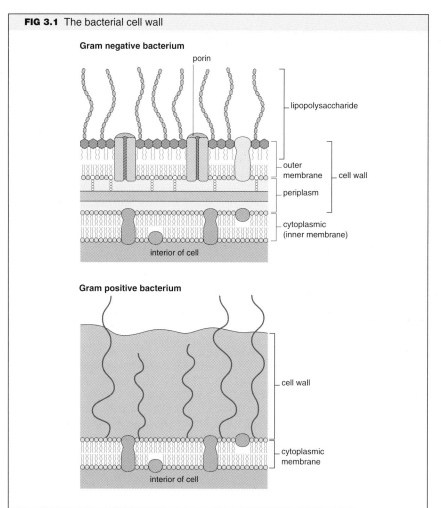

Gram negative bacterium

- porin
- lipopolysaccharide
- outer membrane
- periplasm — cell wall
- cytoplasmic (inner membrane)
- interior of cell

Gram positive bacterium

- cell wall
- cytoplasmic membrane
- interior of cell

TABLE 3.2

Bacterial growth rates (*E. coli*)

Time (h)	No. of bacteria
0	1
1	8
2	64
3	512
4	4096
5	32 768
6	262 144
7	2 097 152
8	16 777 216
9	134 217 728
10	1 073 741 824
11	8 589 934 592
12	68 719 476 736

FIG 3.2 Normal flora of the human body

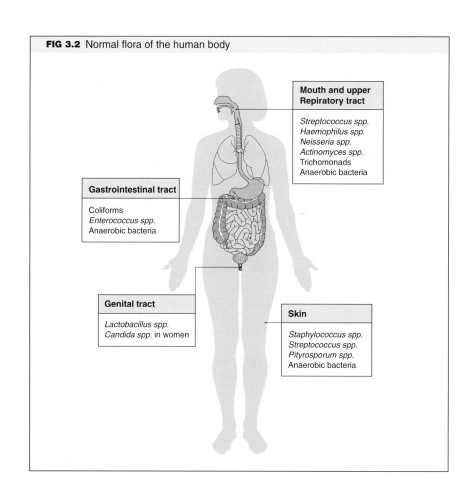

Mouth and upper Repiratory tract

Streptococcus spp.
Haemophilus spp.
Neisseria spp.
Actinomyces spp.
Trichomonads
Anaerobic bacteria

Gastrointestinal tract

Coliforms
Enterococcus spp.
Anaerobic bacteria

Genital tract

Lactobacillus spp.
Candida spp. in women

Skin

Staphylococcus spp.
Streptococcus spp.
Pityrosporum spp.
Anaerobic bacteria

7

4

Fungi — the basic facts

Fungi are eukaryotic organisms that comprise **yeasts, moulds** (filamentous fungi) and **higher fungi** (mushrooms and toadstools). They are widely distributed in the environment and can survive in extreme conditions where nutrients are limited. Most fungi are **saprophytes** (living off dead organic matter) in soil and water and are vital to the carbon cycle. Certain fungi are also of great commercial value in the production of bread, alcohol and antibiotics.

Yeasts are the simplest of the fungi. They are unicellular, spherical in shape and reproduce by budding (**Fig. 4.1**). In some yeasts, including the medically important genus *Candida*, the buds elongate to form filaments (**pseudohyphae**).

Moulds are composed of numerous microscopic branching, filamentous **hyphae**, known collectively as **mycelia**, that are involved in gaining nutrients and reproduction. The reproductive mycelia produce spores, termed **conidia**, either by asexual or sexual reproduction from opposite mating strains. Spores are disseminated in the atmosphere, enabling fungi to colonise new environments.

Certain pathogenic fungi are **dimorphic**, being a yeast form when invading tissues but a mould when living in the environment. The exception is *Candida*, which forms pseudohyphae when in the body.

Diseases caused by fungi

The study of fungi is called **mycology**, and the diseases they cause, **mycoses**. Mycoses are classified depending on the degree of tissue involvement and mode of entry into the host (**Table 4.1**):

- **superficial** — localised to the epidermis, hair and nails but can extend deeper into keratinised tissue
- **subcutaneous** — confined to the dermis, subcutaneous tissue or adjacent structures
- **systemic** — deep infections of the internal organs caused by:
  - **primary pathogenic fungi** that infect previously healthy persons
  - **opportunistic fungi** of marginal pathogenicity that infect the immunocompromised host.

Superficial mycoses These are the most common mycoses of humans and are acquired from the environment, infected humans or natural animal hosts.

Pityriasis versicolor is an infection of the superficial skin and hair which is prevalent in the tropics. Fungi that invade deeper into keratinised cells are termed **dermatophytes**. These diseases are often called **tinea** or **ringworm** because of the characteristic red inflammation with central clearing that forms at the site of infection. Dermatophyte infection affects various sites: e.g. scalp (tinea capitis), foot (tinea pedis: 'athletes foot') and groin (tinea cruris). Although becoming less common, tinea pedis is still the most common fungal infection in the United Kingdom.

Yeast infections are most commonly caused by *Candida albicans* and are confined to the vagina, mouth and soft skin (**candidiasis** or **'thrush'**). A **commensal** of the vagina and gastrointestinal tract, the organism can flourish if ill health, impaired immunity or antibiotic treatment alter the normal bacterial flora.

Subcutaneous mycoses These are infections caused by a number of different fungi that arise from injury to the skin. They usually involve the dermis, subcutaneous tissues and muscle. The fungi commonly live saprophytically on thorn bushes, roses and tree bark, from which wounds can occur. Certain occupational groups (e.g. florists and agricultural workers) are more at risk from infection. Such mycoses are difficult to treat and may require surgical intervention.

Systemic (deep) mycoses These are life-threatening invasive infections caused by a variety of fungi.

The **primary pathogenic fungi** infect previously healthy persons and are caused by **dimorphic** fungi normally found in soil. Infection usually arises from inhaling spores, and the lungs are the main site of infection. However, dissemination to other organs and the central nervous system can occur. The incidence is largely confined to endemic areas in North and South America.

The **opportunistic fungi** infect persons who, usually, have some serious immune or metabolic defect, are on broad-spectrum antibiotics or immunosuppressive drugs, or have undergone major surgery.

Other fungi-related diseases

Certain fungi may indirectly cause human infections. Constant exposure to fungal spores in the atmosphere can induce respiratory allergies, particularly among certain occupational groups (e.g. Farmer's lung). Some mushrooms and toadstools cause poisoning if ingested. Certain moulds produce toxic secondary metabolites (**mycotoxins**) that can contaminate food.

Diagnosis and treatment

The diagnosis and treatment of common mycoses and related diseases is by microscopy and culture of lesions or serology. Antifungal agents are discussed elsewhere.

TABLE 4.1

Common human mycoses

Mycosis	Fungi	Type	Main infection	Epidemiology
Superficial: epidermis, hair and nails but can extend deeper into keratinised tissue	*Candida albicans*	Dimorphic	Oral thrush; vaginitis; cutaneous candidiasis	World-wide
	Malassezia furfur	Dimorphic	Pityriasis versicolor: brown discoloration of the skin	World-wide, especially tropics
	Dermatophytes: *Trichophyton, Microsporum, Epidermophyton*	Filamentous	Tinea (ringworm): skin, hair, nails	World-wide
Subcutaneous: arise from injury to skin and contamination with organic matter	*Sporothrix schenckii*	Dimorphic	Sporotrichosis: ulcerative skin lesion progressing along the lymphatics	World-wide; common in soil and vegetable matter
Systemic — primary pathogenic fungi: internal infections in previously healthy persons	*Histoplasma capsulatum*	Dimorphic	Histoplasmosis: lung lesions (similar to those seen in tuberculosis) spreading into reticuloendothelial system and other organs	North and South America
	Blastomyces dermatitidis	Dimorphic	Blastomycosis: primarily in lung but can spread to skin, bone, viscera and meninges	Eastern parts of USA, Canada, Africa
	Coccidioides immitis	Dimorphic	Coccidioidomycosis: lung lesions leading to generalised tuberculosis-like illness	South-western USA
	Paracoccidioides brasiliensis	Dimorphic	Paracoccidioidomycosis: nasopharynx and lung, with spread to lymphatics	South America (especially Brazil)
Systemic — opportunistic fungi: disseminated infections in the immunocompromised host	*Aspergillus fumigatus*	Filamentous	Invasive aspergillosis; aspergilloma (fungal mass in lungs)	World-wide
	Candida albicans	Dimorphic	Candidiasis	World-wide
	Cryptococcus neoformans	Yeast	Cryptococcosis: can also occur in immunocompetent	World-wide
	Pneumocystis carinii	Yeast-like[a]	Pneumocystis pneumonia	World-wide
Fungal related: allergic reaction; mycotoxin contamination; poisoning by ingestion	**Allergic reactions** *Aspergillus*		Allergic rhinitis, asthma	World-wide
	Alternaria			
	Cladosporium			
	Penicillium			
	Aspergillus fumigatus		Allergic bronchopulmonary aspergillosis	World-wide
	Aspergillus clavatus		Malt workers' lung (extrinsic allergic alveolitis), an occupational disease	World-wide
	Various fungal spores		Sick building syndrome: extrinsic allergic alveolitis often via air conditioning units	World-wide
	Mycotoxins e.g. *Claviceps purpurea*		Ergotism ('madness'): from bread made with rye infected with fungal mycotoxin	World-wide but now rare
	Poisoning e.g. *Amanita phalloides* ('Death cap' mushroom)		Nausea, vomiting, bronchospasm, bradycardia, hallucination, collapse	World-wide

[a]*Pneumocystis carinii* is an intracellular organism, with a life cycle of trophozoite and cyst. Formerly considered to be a protozoan, DNA and RNA sequence analysis have established that it is related to the yeasts.

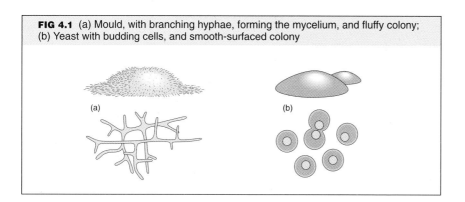

FIG 4.1 (a) Mould, with branching hyphae, forming the mycelium, and fluffy colony; (b) Yeast with budding cells, and smooth-surfaced colony

Protozoa — the basic facts

5

Protozoa, from the Greek meaning 'first animal', refers to simple, **eukaryotic** organisms composed of a microscopic single cell. Reproduction is through simple asexual cell division, or **binary fission**, in which two daughter cells are formed or, if many daughter cells are formed, **multiple fission**. Certain protozoa have complex life cycles involving both asexual (**schizogony**) and sexual reproduction. Some protozoa form resistant cysts that can survive in the environment.

There are over 65 000 known species of protozoa, of which approximately 10 000 are **parasites**, deriving nourishment and environmental protection from inhabiting a living animal host. However, the majority of parasites are non-pathogenic, living as harmless **commensals** within the host. Some animals can harbour parasites and serve as reservoirs for human disease. Infections that are naturally transmitted between animals and humans are termed **zoonoses**. These may be acquired either by direct contact with an animals or indirectly through the ingestion of contaminated water and food. Some zoonoses are spread by the bite of an insect, termed a **vector** in which part of the organism's life cycle is completed.

Only a small number of protozoa cause human disease but those that do affect millions of people world-wide, causing considerable suffering, mortality and economic hardship. Protozoal diseases are largely confined to countries with poor economic and social structure. However, trichomoniasis, crytosporidiosis, and toxoplasmosis are common in developed countries. Protozoa of medical importance are summarised in **Table 5.1**.

The pathogenic protozoa are part of the subkingdom *Protozoa*. Those of medical importance are placed in the phyla *Sarcomastigophora*, *Apicomplexa* and *Ciliophora*. Within these phyla the protozoa are divided into four major classes based on their locomotive form: the amoebae (*Sarcodina*), the flagellates (*Mastigophora*), the sporozoa, and the ciliates (*Kinetofragminophorea*). Examples of common pathogenic protozoa are shown in **Fig. 5.1**.

Amoebae These are the simplest of the protozoa and are characterised by a feeding and dividing trophozoite stage that moves by temporary extensions of the cell called **pseudopodia** ('false feet'). In some species the trophozoite can form a resistant **cyst** stage able to survive in the environment. Those that infect the gut are true parasites being unable to reproduce except in a living host. Others occur naturally in soil and water and are not true parasites. They are termed 'free-living' and infect humans as opportunistic pathogens.

Flagellates These organisms have a trophozoite form but also possess flagella for locomotion and food gathering. All pathogenic species are true parasites, being unable to reproduce outside the host.

Ciliates These possess rows of hair-like cilia around the outside of the body for motility and also to direct food into a primitive mouth termed a cytostome. All ciliates possess two nuclei: a large polyploid micronucleus and a small micronucleus active only during sexual reproduction. Some species form cysts.

Apicomplexa This is a unique group lacking any visible means of locomotion. They are all parasitic and most are intracellular, having a life cycle involving both sexual and asexual reproduction. The common feature of all members is the presence of an **apical complex** (visible only be electron microscopy) at the anterior pole in one or more stages of the life cycle. The exact components of the apical complex vary among members. Its function is thought to enable cell penetration.

Diagnosis and treatment The relatively large size of the protozoa enables most human pathogens to be easily identified by microscopic examination of clinical material. Those of the gut are observed in freshly taken faecal samples. Blood and tissue protozoa are visualised after staining. Detection of elevated antibodies to the infecting organism may be diagnostic in some instances (e.g. toxoplasmosis). Culture methods are not routinely used, as they are technically demanding and time consuming: an exception is the diagnosis of trichomoniasis.

Antiprotozoal therapy is generally unsatisfactory. Treatment is hampered by lack of effective agents for many diseases, their potential toxicity to humans and inability to destroy all forms of the organism. The emergence of drug resistance has also limited the therapeutic potential of many agents.

TABLE 5.1

Common protozoal infections of humans

Organism	Disease and site of infection	Mode of transmission	Geographic distribution
Amoebae			
Entamoeba histolytica	Amoebiasis: gut and occasionally liver	Faecal-oral ingestion of cysts	World-wide
Acanthamoeba	Chronic encephalitis in immunocompromised host	Haematogenous spread from skin or lung	World-wide
	Keratitis (infection of cornea)	Contaminated contact lenses or eye trauma	World-wide
Naegleria fowleri	Acute meningoencephalitis	Nasal instillation whilst swimming	World-wide
Flagellates			
Trichomonas vaginalis	Trichomoniasis: vagina and urethra	Sexually transmitted (usually asymptomatic in males)	World-wide
Giardia lamblia	Giardiasis: gut	Faecal-oral ingestion of cysts	World-wide
Trypanosoma gambiense and *T. rhodesiense*	African trypanosomiasis ('sleeping sickness'): general febrile illness, drowsiness, coma, death	Bite of tsetse fly (*Glossina*): a zoonosis from domestic and wild animals	West Africa: *T. gambiense* East Africa *T. rhodesiense*
Trypanosoma cruzii	American trypanosomiasis ('Chagas' disease'): swelling at bite site (chagoma), fever, lymphadenopathy, hepatosplenomegaly, heart disease, death	Triatomid bug faeces which enters bite wound: a zoonosis from domestic and wild animals	Mexico, Central and South America
Leishmania tropica and *L. major*	Cutaneous leishmaniasis: skin sores	Bite of sandfly (*Phlebotomus*)	Mediterranean, Middle East, North Africa, India, USSR
L. mexicana and *L. braziliensis*	Mucocutaneous leishmaniasis: nose, mouth and palate destruction	Bite of sandfly (*Phlebotomus*)	Mexico, Central and South America
Leishmania donovani	Visceral leishmaniasis ('kala-azar'): liver, spleen, bone marrow and other organs	Bite of sandfly (*Phlebotomus*)	As for other *Leishmania* species
Ciliates			
Balantidium coli	Balantidiosis: gut necrosis, ulceration, bloody diarrhoea; may be asymptomatic	Faecal-oral ingestion of cyts; pigs common reservoir	Russia, northern Europe, North and South America and Asia
Apicomplexa			
Plasmodium falciparum, P. vivax, P. ovale and *P. malariae*	Malaria: liver and erythrocyte infection	Female *Anopheles* mosquito	Africa, Asia and Latin America
Cryptosporidium parvum	Cryptosporidiosis: gut; mild diarrhoea but severe and chronic in immunocompromised	Faecal-oral ingestion of oocysts	World-wide
Toxoplasma gondii	Toxoplasmosis: in immunocompetent — asymptomatic or flu-like symptoms; in immunocompromised — myocarditis, retinochoroiditis, meningoencephalitis, death Congenital infection: retinochoroiditis, hydrocephalus, intracerebral calcification	Ingestion of oocysts from cat faeces; consumption of undercooked meat; transplacental transmission; organ transplantation	World-wide

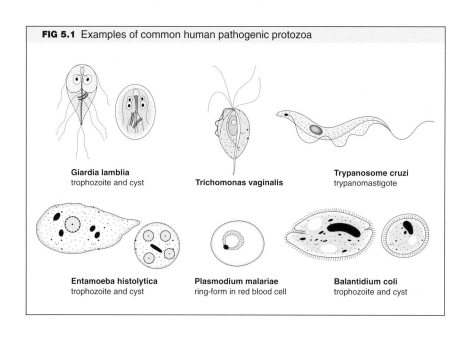

FIG 5.1 Examples of common human pathogenic protozoa

Giardia lamblia
trophozoite and cyst

Trichomonas vaginalis

Trypanosome cruzi
trypanomastigote

Entamoeba histolytica
trophozoite and cyst

Plasmodium malariae
ring-form in red blood cell

Balantidium coli
trophozoite and cyst

11

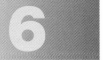

Helminths — the basic facts

Helminths (from the Greek *helminthos*, meaning worm) refers to all parasitic worms of humans. They are complex, multicellular organisms, ranging in size from the microscopic filarial parasites to the giant tapeworms, several metres in length. Sexual reproduction occurs in all cases, usually by mating between male and female larvae. However, some helminths are **hermaphroditic**, possessing both male and female reproductive organs, and can reproduce by self-fertilisation, termed **parthenogenesis**.

Human helminth diseases occur world-wide but are most prevalent in countries with poor socio-economic development. They seldom cause acute disease but produce chronic infections that can have a severely debilitating effect on the host (see **Appendix 5**, p. 129).

Parasitic helminths comprise the **nematodes** (roundworms, filaria), **cestodes** (tapeworms) and **trematodes** (flukes) (**Figs 6.1 and 6.2**).

Nematodes These are typically worm-like in appearance and have the following characteristics:

- They possess a mouth, digestive tract, anus and sexual organs.
- They occur as male or female forms.
- They reproduce by mating or through parthenogenesis of hermaphroditic forms.

The intestinal pathogenic nematodes may be divided into those that develop in the soil (larvae being the infectious stage) and those that do not (eggs are the infectious stage):

- *Development in soil — larvae being infective.* The larvae are shed in the faeces and mature in the soil. They infect humans by burrowing into the skin (usually through the soles of the feet) and enter the blood stream to be carried to the heart and lungs. They then force their way into the alveolus and trachea, and, on reaching the epiglottis, are swallowed. The life cycle then continues in the small intestine.
- *Survival in soil — eggs being infective.* The eggs are the infectious form in which the larvae develop. When ingested the larvae hatch in the small intestine, penetrate the mucosa and are carried through the blood stream to the heart and lungs. The rest of the life cycle is as described above.

In other nematodes the eggs hatch in the intestine where the worms develop and produce eggs that are shed in the faeces. The larvae can sometimes migrate through the body to infect other organs.

Filaria The filaria are microscopic nematodes, transmitted by biting insect **vectors** in which part of the organism's life cycle is completed. On infecting humans the larvae mate and the females produce **microfilariae** which develop in the blood, lymphatic system, skin and eye. This can result in gross swelling of infected tissues, most notably in the groin and legs.

Cestodes (tapeworms) The tapeworms are flat, ribbon-like worms that can grow up to 10 metres in length. They produce eggs which are excreted into the environment and can infect a variety of hosts in which the life cycle continues. Humans become infected from consuming contaminated meat. They are characterised by:

- absent mouth, digestive tract and vascular system
- a **scolex** (head) that attaches to the intestinal wall by suckers
- a **tegument** (body) of the scolex through which nutrients are absorbed
- **proglottids** (segments) forming the tegument, each containing male and female reproductive organs producing infective eggs
- eggs that hatch in the gut, releasing motile larvae that migrate through the gut wall and blood vessels to encyst in muscle forming **cysticerci** (fluid-filled cysts each containing a **scolex**).

Trematodes (flukes) The trematodes are flat, leaf-like organisms. They have complicated life cycles, alternating between a sexual reproductive cycle in the final host (man) and an asexual multiplicative cycle in a snail host. They cause infection of the liver, bladder and rectum. Their major features are:

- They possess a mouth and digestive tract but no anus.
- They are hermaphroditic, except for the schistosomes which have a boat-shaped male and a cylindrical female form.
- Part of their life cycle is completed in an aquatic snail host.

Diagnosis and treatment Intestinal helminths are identified by microscopic examination of faeces. Filaria are detected in blood and tissue samples after staining. As with the protozoa, helminth infections are difficult to treat, because of the lack of effective agents. Those that are available are toxic and unable to destroy all the biological forms (see Chapter 44).

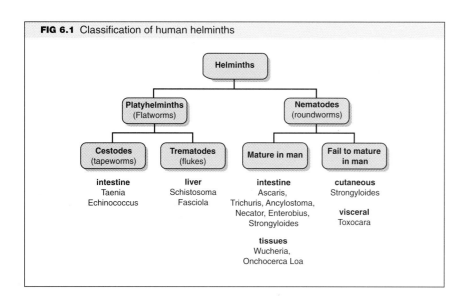

FIG 6.1 Classification of human helminths

Helminths

Platyhelminths (Flatworms)

Nematodes (roundworms)

Cestodes (tapeworms)

Trematodes (flukes)

Mature in man

Fail to mature in man

intestine
Taenia
Echinococcus

liver
Schistosoma
Fasciola

intestine
Ascaris,
Trichuris, Ancylostoma,
Necator, Enterobius,
Strongyloides

tissues
Wucheria,
Onchocerca Loa

cutaneous
Strongyloides

visceral
Toxocara

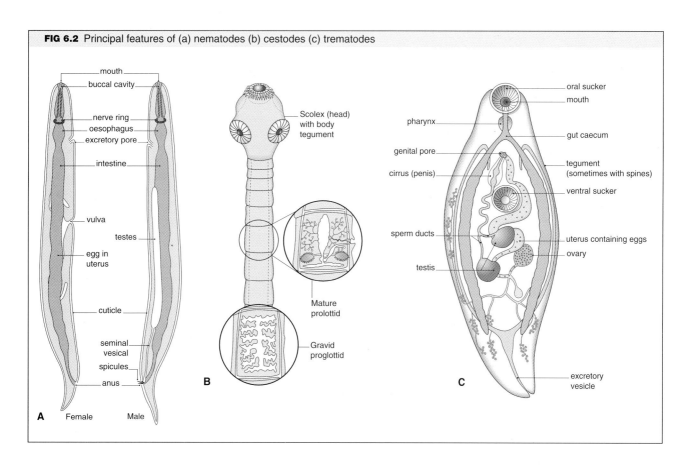

FIG 6.2 Principal features of (a) nematodes (b) cestodes (c) trematodes

A
- mouth
- buccal cavity
- nerve ring
- oesophagus
- excretory pore
- intestine
- vulva
- testes
- egg in uterus
- cuticle
- seminal vesical
- spicules
- anus

Female   Male

B
- Scolex (head) with body tegument
- Mature prolottid
- Gravid proglottid

C
- oral sucker
- mouth
- pharynx
- gut caecum
- genital pore
- cirrus (penis)
- tegument (sometimes with spines)
- ventral sucker
- sperm ducts
- uterus containing eggs
- ovary
- testis
- excretory vesicle

7

Viroids, prions and virinos

These infectious agents are simpler than viruses. Viroids cause, predominantly, plant diseases such as potato spindle-tuber disease. They consist of circular, single-stranded RNA, usually 250 to 370 nucleotides long. In plants they are found mainly in the nucleolus, but little else is known of the pathogenic mechanisms that they employ. Human disease due to viroids is not yet recognised.

Prions are putative infectious agents so-called because they are *pro*teinaceous *in*fectious particles (the originator changed it from proin). Although there is not universal agreement that they exist in vivo, the evidence for them is now considerable. The best studied is the prion that causes a degenerative disorder of the central nervous system of sheep, scrapie. This agent appears to be a 33–35 kDa hydrophobic protein which has been termed PrP (for prion protein). The gene that encodes for this protein exists in normal sheep, but the product in diseased animals has a mutant peptide sequence and an abnormal isoform with β-pleated sheets replacing α-helical domains; the normal cellular protein is termed PrPc, the abnormal PrPsc. The abnormal protein further differs from the normal cellular protein by being insoluble in detergents, highly resistant to proteases and having a tendency to aggregate. Prion proteins have been shown to be infectious and to have a high but not absolute degree of species specificity.

An alternative hypothesis for the infectious agent of scrapie has been the **virino**. This putative agent has a tiny, as yet undetectable, scrapie-specific nucleic acid coated in PrP. There is currently no evidence for the existence of this agent, but it offers a plausible explanation for the strain variation that is known to occur in scrapie.

Transmissible degenerative encephalopathies
Scrapie is a transmissible degenerative encephalopathy (TDE) of sheep, and many other ungulates suffer this disorder (**Table 7.1**). It is now recognised that TDEs also occur in man (**Table 7.2**). The features of a TDE are:

- the presence of aggregates of prion proteins into amyloid fibrils
- the presence of 'holes' in the neuronal matrix ('spongiform' degeneration) caused by amyloid (**Fig. 7.1**)
- a long incubation period (several months to many years)
- that they are rapidly progressive
- clinical presentation with cognitive impairment, ataxia, myoclonus and extrapyramidal signs.

The tentative diagnosis of human TDE is made from the clinical features, which occur usually in patients between 40 and 70 years of age; 'variant' Creutzfeld–Jakob (vCJD) disease, however, involves younger patients. Confirmation of the diagnosis currently depends on the neuropathological features found at post-mortem, although newer methods based on detection of the abnormal PrP by labelled-specific antibody are becoming more widely available and constitute the definitive test. Currently there is no treatment, so prevention forms the bedrock of control. Brain and spinal cord appear to be the predominant reservoir of infection, and transmission has been shown to occur with infected corneal and dura mater grafts, growth hormone and gonadotrophin injections and the use of contaminated neurosurgical instruments. Kuru is thought to have arisen because of cannibalism of human brains. There is also a genetic component to disease susceptibility, with 10% of CJD cases being familial and a higher prevalence of sporadic CJD in, for example, Israeli Jews of Libyan origin. The human prion protein gene is located on chromosome 20, and homozygosity at codon 129 (methionine or valine) confers susceptibility to CJD, although this mutation is not directly linked to disease causation. Such markers may be useful in the future for diagnostic and screening purposes.

TABLE 7.1

Transmissible degenerative encephalopathies of animals

Disease	Host
Scrapie	Sheep, goats
Bovine spongiform encephalopathy (BSE)	Cattle
Feline spongiform encephalopathy (FSE)	Cats
Transmissible mink encephalopathy (TME)	Mink
Chronic wasting disease (CWD)	Mule deer, elk
Exotic ungulate encephalopathy (EUE)	Nyala, greater kudu

TABLE 7.2

Human prion diseases

Disease	Notes
Creutzfeld–Jakob disease (CJD)	Can be iatrogenic, sporadic or familial. Iatrogenic cases have mean incubation periods from 18 months for intracerebral inoculation by contaminated neurosurgical instruments to 13 years from the use of contaminated gonadotrophin given parenterally
Gerstmann–Straussler–Scheinker (GSS) syndrome	Familial. Rare. Progression is usually slower than in CJD with characteristic multicentric amyloid plaques in the brains of all cases
Kuru	Disease described in the Fore tribe of Papua–New Guinea. No new cases since 1957 when cannibalism was stopped
Fatal familial insomnia (FFI)	Familial. Rare. Originally described in Italian families with selective neuropathology in the thalamus
Variant Creutzfeld–Jakob disease (vCJD)	First described in 1996. Strongly linked to ingestion of BSE-contaminated meat products. Occurs in young and older adults. Neuropathology shows more severe spongiform change in cerebellum and cerebral cortex than 'classic' CJD. Has only been described in the UK

FIG 7.1a Histology of spongiform degeneration — spongiform degeneration in CJD

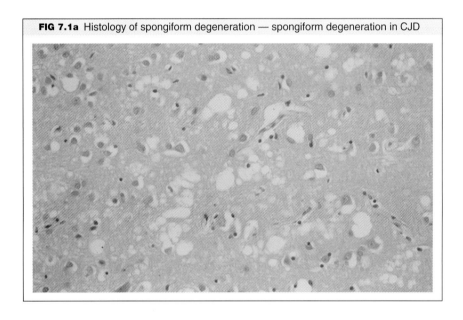

FIG 7.1b Histology of spongiform degeneration — prion protein staining of CJD brain tissue

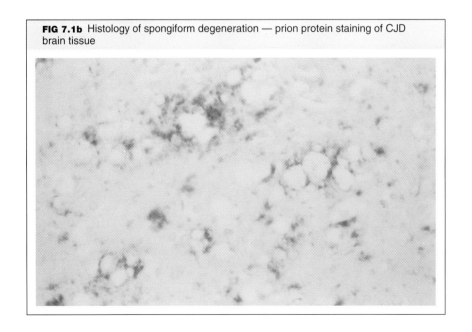

SAQ 1 — Basic microbiology

Questions

1. List four differences between prokaryotes and eukaryotes.

2. What is meant by the following terms when applied to the classification of bacteria: taxonomy, biovars, strains, serovars, phylogeny?

3. Describe the differences between rickettsias, chlamydiae and other bacteria.

4. What is the Lancefield grouping system, α-haemolysis and β-haemolysis?

5. List two Gram-positive human pathogens which form endospores.

6. What are the taxonomic differences in the terms '*Herpesviridae*', '*Alphaherpesvirinae*' and '*Simplexvirus*'?

7. Order the following viruses in descending order of size: influenza virus, parvovirus B19, rhinovirus, vaccinia virus.

8. Name three medically important dimorphic fungi.

9. Draw a simple diagram of the structure of an amoeba, labelling the parts.

10. Draw a flow chart of the life cycle of human schistosomes.

Answers

1. Protozoa, helminths, fungi and higher plants and animals consist of eukaryotic cells (from Greek for 'good nut', the nut referring to the nucleus). Bacteria are prokaryotes. Differences are:

   - Eukaryotes have a nuclear membrane.
   - Eukaryotes have cytoplasmic organelles.
   - Eukaryotes have a cytoskeleton.
   - Eukaryotes possess a nucleolus.
   - Eukaryotic DNA is present in a complex with histones.
   - Eukaryotes have more than one chromosome.
   - Eukaryotic cells undergo mitosis.
   - Eukaryotic ribosomes are 80S (except in mitochondria and chloroplasts), prokaryotic ribosomes are 70S.
   - Eukaryotes mostly lack an external cell wall; if present it is of different chemical composition to prokaryotic cell walls.
   - Eukaryotic flagella and cilia have a 9+2 pattern of microtubules.

2. **Taxonomy** (from the Greek for 'govern arrangement') is the science of biological classification, consisting of organising organisms into groups or taxa. **Biovars** are variant bacterial species with differing biochemical and/or physiological characteristics from the prototype strain. A **strain** is a population of bacteria that descends from a single parent. **Phylogeny** (from the Greek for 'tribe') is the classification based on evolutionary relationships; most commonly this is done by comparing 16S ribosomal RNA sequences. The bible of bacterial classification is *Bergey's Manual of Systematic Bacteriology*.

3. Unlike other bacteria, rickettsias and chlamydiae are Gram-negative organisms which are obligate intracellular parasites: they can only grow and reproduce within host cells. They are smaller, being only a little larger than the largest viruses, and are limited metabolically. Chlamydiae have cell walls deficient in muramic acid and peptidoglycan.

4. These all pertain to the descriptive classification of streptococci and related Gram-positive organisms.

One characteristic of some streptococci is the ability to lyse erythrocytes. When grown on blood agar, β-**haemolysis** is seen when there is complete haemolysis, manifest as a zone of clearing, around the culture; α-**haemolysis** is a green zone due to partial lysis of erythrocytes. The Lancefield system is used to further subdivide β-haemolytic streptococci antigenically.

5. Bacteria can produce **endospores** which allow the organism to survive under extreme conditions, such as desiccation and heat. Gram-positive endospore producers of medical importance are members of the *Bacillus* and *Clostridium* species. Examples are *Bacillus cereus*, a food-poisoning organism, and *Clostridium tetani*, which is responsible for tetanus.

6. Virus terminology does not follow the Linnaean nomenclature. Virus families have the suffix *-viridae*, subfamilies *-virinae* and the genus *-virus*. Thus *Herpesviridae* is a family which contains the subfamily *Alphaherpesvirinae* which, in turn contains the genus *Simplexvirus*. Note that these names are all italicised by convention, but common names such as varicella-zoster virus are not.

7. Human viruses range in size from 20 nm in diameter to over 290 nm. RNA viruses are generally smaller than DNA viruses, with poxviruses, including vaccinia virus, being the largest. The smallest group of DNA viruses, such as parvoviruses are, however, slightly smaller than the smallest RNA viruses, the *Picornaviridae*, which includes rhinoviruses.

8. **Dimorphic fungi** are those that can exist in either yeast or mycelial (mould) form. Examples are: *Candida albicans*, *Coccidioides capsulatum*, *Histoplasma capsulatum*, *Sporothrix schenckii*, *Blastomyces dermatidis*, *Paracoccidioides brasiliensis*.

9. See Figure, p. 120.

10. Protozoa and helminths have complex life cycles, with man only being a part. An example is that of schistosomes. See Figure, p. 120.

Epidemiology of infectious diseases

8

Epidemiology is 'the study of the occurrence, distribution and control of disease in populations'. The risk of infection is not just dependent upon an individual's susceptibility but on the level of disease within the population, the degree of **population mixing** and **herd immunity**, as well as specific features such as the **communicable period**, **route** and ease (**infectiousness**) of transmission.

Route of transmission

For an infectious agent to persist within a population there must be a *cycle* of transmission from a contaminated **source**, through a **portal of entry**, into a susceptible host and on again (**Fig. 8.1**):

- **Direct transmission**, the most common and important route, involves all forms of physical contact between humans, including sexual transmission, faecal-oral spread, and *direct* respiratory spread via large droplets.
- **Vector-borne transmission** is mediated by **arthropods or insects**; it is **mechanical** if the vector is simply a source of contamination, but **biological** if it is necessary for the multiplication or maturation of the infectious agent.
- **Vehicle-borne transmission** describes the spread from all contaminated inanimate objects. Vehicles include clothing, food, water, surgical instruments and also biological substances such as blood and tissues.
- **Airborne transmission** is mediated by aerosols suspended in the air for long periods.
- A **zoonosis** is any infection spread from a vertebrate animal to a human.

Disease in the population

Prevalence is 'the number of cases of infection per unit of population at a single point in time'. **Incidence** refers to 'the number of new cases of infection per unit of population over a specified period of time'. For **acute** infections, lasting only a few days or possibly weeks, the incidence may be very high but the prevalence relatively low. However, for **chronic** infections, lasting months or years, the prevalence may be relatively high even though the incidence is low. Infections like urinary tract infections occur at roughly steady levels throughout the year, although others may vary — for example the rise in respiratory tract infections during the winter. The **periodicity** of some infections is measured over a much longer scale, for example the roughly 4-yearly cycle in mycoplasma pneumonias.

Infections that have a stable incidence within the population are described as **endemic** (or **hyperendemic** if the incidence is extremely high). Cases are frequently unconnected and are therefore referred to as **sporadic**. A number of terms are used to describe situations in which the *number of infections is greater than that which might be anticipated from previous experience*:

- A cluster of cases in a single household or over a small area is described as an **outbreak**. It may relate to exposure to a local source, and suitable detective work and control procedures may prevent further transmission.
- An increase in cases over a larger region, perhaps an entire country, is described as an **epidemic**. This is less likely to be due to a single source, and more extensive measures will be required to control the spread.
- If the increase occurs over a larger area still, for example several countries, it is described as a **pandemic**.

The burden of infectious diseases varies enormously throughout the world (**Table 8.1**), dependent upon factors such as environmental conditions, wealth and nutritional status, local human behaviour and the efficiency of health care. Health service managers clearly need this information to plan for the future; however, it is vital that *every clinician* be aware of regional patterns of disease for the effective diagnosis, treatment and control of infection within their own practice of medicine (**Table 8.2**). For serious communicable diseases in the UK, **surveillance** is achieved through a *legal requirement* for medical practitioners to inform the local 'consultant in communicable disease control' (or the 'consultant in public health medicine' in Scotland) of *all* cases of **notifiable disease** (see Appendix 3). For less serious infections, individual general practices or hospital units may volunteer to report their cases of infection through government or professional association programmes.

TABLE 8.1

Some major world health problems

Disease	Region	Number of cases	Comments
Tuberculosis	World-wide, esp. developing countries	1/3 of the world population infected (50 million multi-drug resistant cases?)	3 million deaths/year
Malaria	Tropical and subtropical regions	300–500 million clinical cases/year	1.5–2.5 million deaths/year
Schistosomiasis	Africa, Latin America & S.E. Asia	200 million infected	20 000 deaths/year
Filariasis	Asia, Africa, Latin America & Pacific Islands	120 million infected	
Infectious diarrhoea	World-wide, esp. developing countries	1500 million cases/year	4 million deaths of children < 5 years
Gonorrhoea	World-wide, esp. developing countries	62 million new cases/year	Infertility; ↑ risk HIV infection; up to 30% neonates → ophthalmia neonatorum
Food-borne trematode infections	Esp. S.E. Asia	40 million infected	>10 000 deaths/year
Measles	World-wide, esp. developing countries	40 million cases/year	Case fatality rate up to 30%
Onchocerciasis	Africa & C. America	18 million infected	270 000 blind
Chagas' disease	C. & S. America	16–18 million infected	45 000 deaths/year
Leishmaniasis	Mostly tropical and subtropical areas	12 million infected	500 000 cases visceral leishmaniasis
Dengue haemorrhagic fever	C. America & S.E. Asia	500 000 hospital cases/year	1000 deaths/year
Neonatal tetanus	Developing countries, esp. Asia	400 000 cases/year	Case fatality rate up to 80%

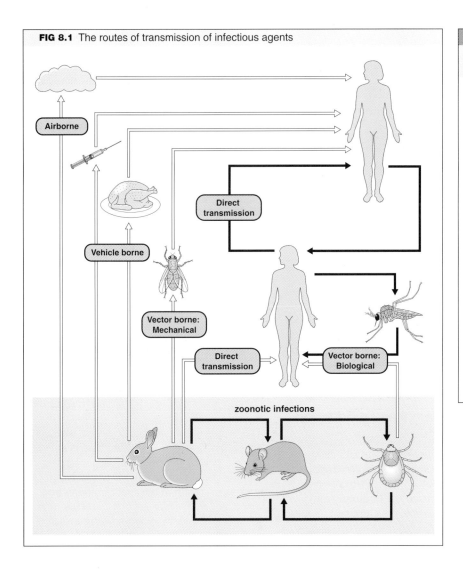

FIG 8.1 The routes of transmission of infectious agents

Airborne

Vehicle borne

Vector borne: Mechanical

Direct transmission

Direct transmission

Vector borne: Biological

zoonotic infections

TABLE 8.2

GP consultation rates per 10 000 person years at risk in UK

Acute respiratory tract infection	4376
Arthropathy, including back pain/rheumatism	2976
'Non-infective' skin disorders	1818
Non-psychotic mental disorders	1466
Hypertension and ischaemic heart disease	1462
Female genital tract disorders, including PID	1139
Contraceptive advice	1119
Eye disease, including infection	866
Vaccination	791
Other 'viral' diseases	687
Superficial fungal infections	617
Upper intestinal tract disorders	584
Cystitis and other urinary tract disorders	565
Intestinal infectious disease	518
Neoplasms	492
Skin / subcutaneous tissue infections	471

9

Pathogenesis of infectious disease

Only a minority of micro-organisms are in contact with humans, and most of these are commensal flora within their own ecological niche. However, viruses and other **pathogenic** micro-organisms characteristically cause disease; they may have highly specific **adhesins** and **toxins**, the genes for which may be grouped together under the control of a single promoter in **pathogenicity islands**. The net result of the meeting between a human and any micro-organism depends on the balance between **host immunity** and the **virulence** of the infectious agent (**Table 9.1** and **Fig. 9.1**). However, interaction with micro-organisms occurs continually, and disease is common — how do we know if the two are linked? **Koch's postulates** (**Table 9.2**) are an important set of criteria that can be used to judge whether a micro-organism is the cause of a disease. They are still relevant today, although it is difficult to apply them to poorly demarcated clinical syndromes: such as diseases where the pathogen that initiated a disease process is no longer present, as occurs in some autoimmune diseases; malignancies; multifactorial diseases; serious diseases without an animal model; infections in the immunocompromised; and uncultivatable micro-organisms.

Contact and adhesion

Infectious agents must gain entry to the host and stick to target tissues.

- Portals of entry include the **gastrointestinal tract, respiratory mucosa, genital mucosa**, and **direct inoculation through the skin.**
- Many agents have **adhesins** on their surface or on **fimbriae** which project from the cell. Parasites may even physically hold on to their host (**Table 9.3**).
- Adhesion will protect micro-organisms from the flushing of mucosal surfaces. Gastrointestinal pathogens have some resistance to gastric acid and bile, whilst agents of skin infections are resistant to drying.

Evasion of host defences / production of virulence factors

Micro-organisms that successfully invade host tissues increase their numbers by producing a range of factors that enable them to survive the onslaught of innate and specific immunity and which are responsible for the development of clinical disease.

- **Toxins (Table 9.4)** are substances that can damage a host's cells and which may be active away from the site of production. An **exotoxin** is secreted, whilst an **endotoxin** is a constitutive part of the pathogen, in particular the **lipopolysaccharide** (LPS) of the Gram-negative bacterial cell wall. Toxins may be subdivided further, for example according to their cellular target, their mode of action or their biological effect. Some toxins, such as TSST-1, have an additional effect of acting as superantigens causing polyclonal activation and cytokine release to impair an effective immune response. If developing T-cells are exposed, deletion of that clone results.
- Other virulence factors may also be produced that tend to be locally acting without causing cellular damage. For example, some *Staphylococcus aureus* strains may produce a **coagulase** that coagulates fibrinogen and increases the likelihood of abscess formation, whilst others may produce a **hyaluronidase** that breaks down intercellular junctions, leading to cellulitis. Different species of bacteria produce different kinases, lecithinases and proteases, which partly explains the range in virulence and clinical presentation of the various agents.
- Other factors include **siderophores** that steal essential iron from host carrier proteins, secreted surface **capsules** that reduce phagocytic efficiency, factors that prevent phagosome lysozome fusion and substances that allow the pathogen to escape from the phagosome into the host cytoplasm.

Transmission

To complete the cycle of infection, infectious agents will need to be excreted, the route dictating the mechanism of spread:

- Faecal-oral spread involves excretion within stool samples and may be aided by the production of copious volumes of hygiene-challenging diarrhoea.
- Pathogens spread via the respiratory tract can be found in respiratory tract secretions, often aerosolised by sneezing and coughing.
- Vaginal/cervical or urethral discharges contain infectious agents that are transmitted by sexual contact.
- The means of transmitting zoonotic infections are diverse for diseases where man is a normal part of the infectious cycle. They include the obvious methods of discharge, such as excretion of the agent in faeces and urine, but also means such as **parasitaemia**, to ensure uptake by blood-sucking insects (e.g. anopholene mosquitos and malaria), and the budding of rabies virus from the apical surfaces of salivary gland epithelia to account for spread via the bite of a rabid animal.

TABLE 9.1

Pathogenesis and definitions

- *contamination*: micro-organism comes into direct contact with the host
- *colonisation*: micro-organism multiplies or develops within the host
- *infectious disease*: micro-organism multiplies or develops within the host *and* produces damage and/or cellular response
- *pathogenicity*: the ability of a micro-organism to cause an infection in the host
- *virulence*: the degree of pathogenicity of a micro-organism
- *commensalism*: 'eating at the same table' — a neutral relationship
- *symbiosis*: mutually beneficial relationship
- *parasitism*: an uneven relationship — one organism benefits at the expense of the other

TABLE 9.2

Koch's postulates

1. The organism occurs in every case of the disease and under circumstances which account for the pathological changes and clinical course of the disease.

2. The organism occurs in no other disease as a fortuitous and non-pathogenic finding.

3. After being isolated from the body and grown in pure culture, the organism will *repeatedly* produce exactly the same clinical disease when inoculated into a new host.

4. The organism can then be isolated from the new host(s).

TABLE 9.3

Infectious agents and adhesion

Non-specific

Infectious agent	Mechanism	
Giardia lamblia	Mechanical 'gripping disc'	
Staphylococcus epidermidis	Polysaccharide slime	
Pseudomonas aeruginosa	Alginate production	

Specific (adhesins)

Infectious agent	Adhesin	Receptor
Entamoeba histolytica	Galactose-binding lectin	Galactose
Escherichia coli (fimbrial)	P fimbriae	Uroepithelial cells; P blood group antigen
Yersinia enterocolitica (non-fimbrial)	Ail protein	Epithelial integrin
Human immunodeficiency virus (HIV)	gp 120	CD4 antigen

TABLE 9.4

Examples of bacterial toxins

Name	Source	Receptor	Biological effect
Cholera toxin	*Vibrio cholerae*	GM1 ganglioside	Activation of adenylate cyclase; secretory diarrhoea
Diphtheria toxin	*Corynebacterium diphtheriae*	EGF-like growth factor precursor	Inhibition of protein synthesis; cell death
Oedema factor	*Corynebacterium anthracis*	Unknown glycoprotein	↑ Target cell cAMP; haemolysis
Shiga toxin	*Shigella dysenteriae*	Globotriaosylcer-amide	↓ Protein synthesis; cell death
Tetanus toxin	*Clostridium tetani*	Ganglioside	↓ Neurotransmitter release; spastic paralysis
TSST-1	*Staphylococcus aureus*	T-cell receptor	'Superantigen', uncoordinated immunological stimulation

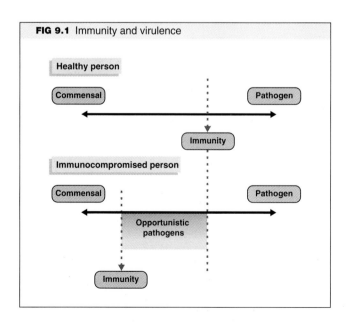

FIG 9.1 Immunity and virulence

Pathology of infectious disease

10

Symptoms of infection arise from direct damage to tissues, 'poisoning of cells', immune-mediated damage (**immunopathology**), or a combination of these. Subclinical infection may occur, however, without any such damage. Disease severity depends on both host factors and virulence determinants of the micro-organism (**Tables 10.1 and 10.2**); even in an outbreak arising from a single pathogen, there is often a spectrum of clinical presentation.

Damage to tissues

Most viruses cause damage to the cells they infect. Viruses abort host replicative mechanisms and may cause death of the cell that way or, when mature, lyse the cell when they erupt. If a large fraction of the cells is infected then there is extensive tissue damage. Programmed cell death, or **apoptosis** is also now recognised as a common mechanism that many viruses, such as HIV and influenza A, use to cause cell damage. Macroscopically, extensive tissue necrosis is, however, rare, and patchy necrosis with oedema due to membrane damage is all that is seen. Viral infection is also characterised by changes in the cytoskeleton and organelles. There may be shrinkage of the nucleus, **pyknosis**, and aggregations of newly formed virus seen as **inclusion bodies**. Some viruses, such as paramyxoviruses, also cause cell-to-cell fusion to yield multinucleate cells.

Viruses such as hepatitis B virus, herpesviruses (particularly EBV) and papillomaviruses are known to be oncogenic. The precise mechanisms of cancer causation are not fully elucidated but genes that provide oncogenic potential are identified: for example the product of the X-gene of hepatitis B virus has been shown to inhibit DNA repair mechanisms and therefore allow the accumulation of mutations.

Bacteria may exist intracellularly within phagocytic cells. These cells may then be destroyed. Parenchymal cells are, however, more commonly damaged by extracellular products such as toxins, enzymes and pH change. *Helicobacter pylori*, for example, produces urease which causes H$^+$ ion changes and mucinase which degrades the protective mucous layer of the stomach cavity; both of these mechanisms are thought to contribute to the cell damage that results in gastritis and peptic ulceration.

Cell toxicity

Viruses can be broadly considered as cell poisons. Bacteria exert most of their direct cell and tissue damage through the production of toxins. The end result tends to be loss of function which might be manifest as oedema and necrosis of tissue, but may not have macroscopic effects. Some fungi can also produce toxins, a well-characterised example being aflatoxin produced by *Aspergillus flavus* which contaminates monkey nuts.

Inflammation and immunopathology

Acute inflammation with an influx of neutrophils and other inflammatory cells can produce obvious changes in the tissue (**Fig. 10.1**). If this is extensive then long-term fibrotic changes may result. Immunopathology can result from different types of immune reaction to infection (**Table 10.3**). The cell-mediated immune response to *Mycobacterium tuberculosis* results in characteristic pathology with granulomata exhibiting central caseous ('cheesy') necrosis (**Fig. 10.2**).

The production of autoantibodies (to DNA, erythrocytes, etc.) is not uncommon, but overt **autoimmune** disease occurs as a result of few infections (**Table 10.4**). Simplistically, these arise because of molecular mimicry between host components and foreign antigens, with an immune response initially directed against an antigen on the microbe then recognising a similar structure of a host component as foreign.

TABLE 10.1

Host determinants of disease severity

- age
- nutritional status
- genetic constitution (race, HLA type, others)
- immune status
- physiology (gastric pH, cilial function, secretions)
- normal flora/hygiene
- presence of physical barriers (intact skin/mucous membranes, absence of foreign bodies)
- antimicrobial usage (may be both a positive and a negative factor)

TABLE 10.2

Microbial determinants of virulence

- infectious dose
- route of infection
- genetics
- expressed virulence factors/aggressins

TABLE 10.3

Immunopathological reactions

Type	Immunopathology	Examples
I	Antigen binds to IgE → mast cell degranulation → release of cytokines → anaphylaxis, allergic type response	Helminth infections, RS virus wheezing
II	Antigen binds to antibody on cell surface → activation of complement/ADCC → cytotoxicity	(?) Fulminant viral hepatitis
III	Antigen binds to free antibody → immune complexes → vasculitis/inflammation	Arthritis in hepatitis B
IV	Antigen reacts with sensitised T cells → delayed cytotoxicity → inflammation/tissue damage	Tuberculosis, leprosy

TABLE 10.4

Examples of autoimmune disease following infections

Disease	Infectious agent
Rheumatic fever	Group A streptococci
Diabetes mellitus	Coxsackie B viruses
Thyroiditis	Enteroviruses
Reactive arthritis	*Chlamydia trachomatis, Salmonella* spp.

FIG 10.1 Bacterial pneumonia showing acute inflammatory response

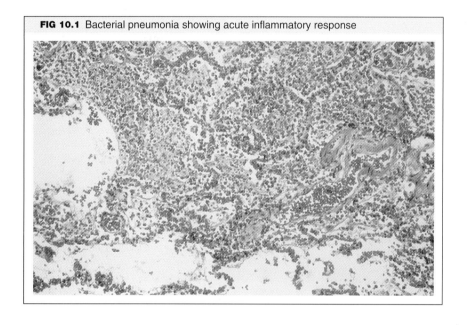

FIG 10.2 Tuberculosis of lymph node, showing caseous necrosis

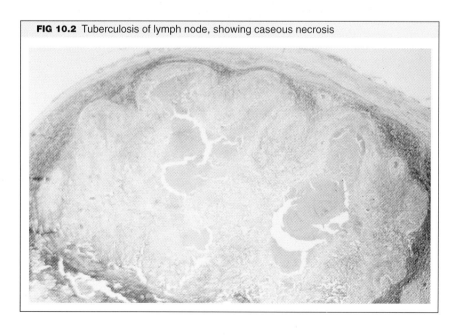

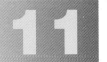

Innate host defences to infectious disease

The skin and mucous membranes are physical barriers that form the first defence against infection (**Fig. 11.1**). They are characterised by high cell turnover, with superficial cells, which may have become colonised by pathogens over time, constantly being shed from the surface. Most sites are further protected by secretions of **mucus**, which trap micro-organisms and prevent them sticking directly to epithelial cells, and substances such as lysozyme (a powerful degradative enzyme) and lactoferrin (an iron-binding protein which makes the essential acquisition of iron by bacteria difficult). Environments may be made more hostile still by an acid **pH**, such as in the stomach, vagina or urine, or by alkaline pH, such as in the duodenum. It is also difficult for micro-organisms to rest on epithelial surfaces, because of the peristalsis of gut contents, periodic flushing of the urethra with urine, and the **muco-ciliary escalator** of the respiratory tract. The normal bacterial flora at many of these sites may also be protective against incoming pathogens because of:

- scavenging of all available nutrients
- the maintenance of hostile conditions, e.g. the metabolic activity of *Lactobacillus* spp. contributes to the acid pH of the vagina
- natural production of 'antibiotics'
- ensuring 'fitness' of specific immunity by subclinical stimulation at mucosal sites.

Within tissues there is a series of **phagocytic cells** that ingest micro-organisms into **phagosomes**, which then merge with intracytoplasmic granules (**lysosomes**) containing toxic reagents to form **phagolysosomes**, where the micro-organisms will be killed by **oxygen-dependent** and **oxygen-independent** mechanisms (**Fig. 11.2**). These **antigen-presenting cells** then channel the breakdown products from the phagocytosed micro-organisms onto their surface, where they are made available for stimulation of passing cells from the specific immune system. **Natural killer** cells are cytotoxic cells; they are related to T lymphocytes, but as they act non-specifically and without memory they are included here.

A number of **acute-phase proteins** are produced in response to infection, including the **complement system**. This describes a series of proteins that are sequentially activated, with some of the later products of the cascade amplifying the activation of earlier components through **positive feedback**. The process may be initiated directly by contact with micro-organisms (the **alternative** and **mannan-binding lectin** pathways) or through the recognition of antibody–antigen complexes (the **classic** pathway). However, the later stages of the cascade and the net results are the same regardless of the mechanism of activation. Complement factors are either deposited onto the surface of micro-organisms or liberated into the site of infection with the following effects:

- **Inflammation**: some products are **chemotactic** factors that attract more cells of the immune system to the area.
- **Opsonisation**: some factors, when deposited on the surface of micro-organisms, improve the efficiency of phagocytic uptake.
- **Lysis:** the terminal components of the complement system form a ring-like structure on the surface of infectious agents which punches a hole in the membrane, leading to death of the cell.

Although it is possible to identify the above elements as providing **innate** or **non-specific** immunity, in practice they will act in conjunction with parts of the **adaptive immune system**. For example, antigen presentation by phagocytes is essential for T helper cell stimulation; in turn, antibody can act as an opsonin, and **cytokine** production by activated T helper cells turns on oxygen-dependent killing, both of which improve the efficiency of phagocytosis. Cytokines (**Table 11.1**) are soluble mediators that produce complex overlapping signals between the host's cells; they are secreted by **monocytes, macrophages** and **lymphocytes** and other cells. Those that are responsible for communication between cells of the immune system are called **interleukins**. Cytokines such as IL-1, IL-6 and IFN-α mainly promote non-specific immunity, whilst IL-2 mainly affects cells of the specific immune system. TNF and IFN-γ tend to increase inflammation, whilst GM-CSF targets precursor cells within the bone marrow. Most cytokines have a stimulatory effect, but IL-10 tends to suppress immune function. There are over two hundred cytokines now recognised, but the role of most in the host defence to infection has yet to be established.

TABLE 11.1

Source and effects of some selected cytokines

Cytokine	Source	Target	Action
Interleukin-1 (IL-1)	Macrophages	Lymphocytes	General activation
		Phagocytes	General activation
		Hepatocytes	Synthesis of acute-phase proteins
Interleukin-6 (IL-6)	Macrophages & CD4+ T cells	B lymphocytes	Differentiation & antibody secretion
		Hepatocytes	Synthesis of acute-phase proteins
Interferon-α (IFN-α)	Monocytes	T lymphocytes	Increases natural killer activity
		Infected cells	Increased HLA I expression & inhibition of viral replication
Tumour necrosis Factor (TNF)	T lymphocytes	Lymphocytes	General activation
	Monocytes	Phagocytes	General activation
		Hepatocytes	Synthesis of acute-phase proteins
Interleukin-2 (IL-2)	CD4+ T lymphocytes	T lymphocytes	Proliferation and maturation
		Natural killer cells	Activation
Interferon-γ (IFN-γ)	T lymphocytes	Macrophages	Activation
		Most tissues	Increased HLA Class I and II expression
Granulocyte/macrophage-colony stimulating factor (GM-CSF)	T cells, macrophages, endothelial cells, macrophages	Granulocytes & monocytes	Increased growth and differentiation of precursors
Interleukin-10 (IL-10)	Lymphocytes & macrophages	T cells & macrophages	Inhibits cytokine production
		Antigen presenting cells	Decreases HLA class II expression

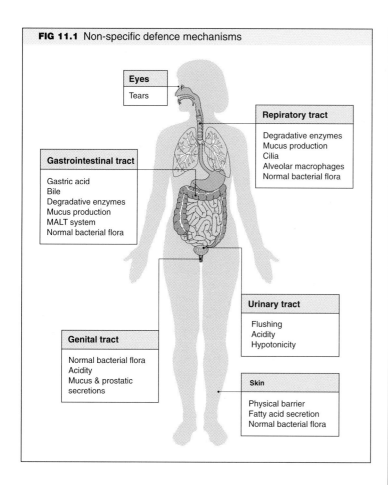

FIG 11.1 Non-specific defence mechanisms

Eyes

Tears

Repiratory tract

Degradative enzymes
Mucus production
Cilia
Alveolar macrophages
Normal bacterial flora

Gastrointestinal tract

Gastric acid
Bile
Degradative enzymes
Mucus production
MALT system
Normal bacterial flora

Urinary tract

Flushing
Acidity
Hypotonicity

Genital tract

Normal bacterial flora
Acidity
Mucus & prostatic
secretions

Skin

Physical barrier
Fatty acid secretion
Normal bacterial flora

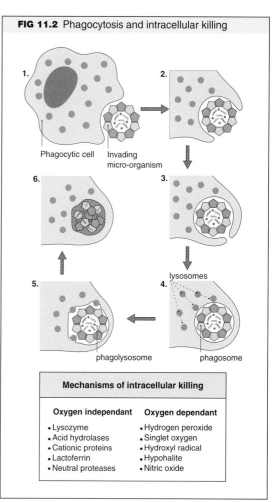

FIG 11.2 Phagocytosis and intracellular killing

1.

Phagocytic cell   Invading micro-organism

2.

6.

3.

5.

lysosomes

4.

phagolysosome   phagosome

Mechanisms of intracellular killing

Oxygen independant	Oxygen dependant
• Lysozyme	• Hydrogen peroxide
• Acid hydrolases	• Singlet oxygen
• Cationic proteins	• Hydroxyl radical
• Lactoferrin	• Hypohalite
• Neutral proteases	• Nitric oxide

12 Adaptive host response to infectious disease

In contrast to innate immunity, **acquired, adaptive** or **specific immunity** is both highly specific in its recognition of foreign material and also becomes more efficient with repeated exposure to the same micro-organism. The pivotal cell is the **lymphocyte**, which is able to respond to a *single* foreign **antigen**. This clearly requires a massive number of cells if an individual is to be able to react to the huge range of micro-organisms that may be encountered in a lifetime. This diversity is generated by having multiple, variable germ line genes coding for antigen receptors that recombine in a random manner within each precursor lymphocyte; these cells then mature in early life, by a process of **positive** and **negative selection**, to give a mixed population of competent cells that can be activated but which will not react against 'self'. Upon exposure to the appropriate antigen they proliferate and differentiate either into short-acting 'effector' cells or into long-lasting memory cells that allow a more rapid and greater response on subsequent exposure to the *same* antigen (**Fig. 12.1**). Lymphocytes may usefully be divided up into: **B lymphocytes (humoral immunity)** and **T lymphocytes (cell-mediated immunity)**; according to the molecules that they express on their surface, e.g. **Cluster Differentiation** (CD) markers; and by their pattern of cytokine production, e.g. Th1 v Th2 v Th0 cells (**Fig. 12.2**).

Each B lymphocyte has **antibodies** or **immunoglobulins**, specific for just one antigen, arranged facing outwards as receptors on its surface; if exposed to that antigen, the B cell proliferates and then differentiates (**Fig. 12.1**). Its effectors are called **plasma cells**, and each one can only produce antibody of *single* antigen specificity, although the **isotype** may vary as the immune response matures. The basic structure of an antibody is shown in **Fig. 12.3**, with the various isotypes described in **Table 12.1**. The

pattern of antibody production demonstrates the importance of memory in increasing the speed and strength of response with secondary exposure, and also the effect of **isotype switching**, as IgM is only produced in primary infection (**Fig. 12.4**). Antibodies are important for:

- **complement activation** (initiation of the classic pathway via the Fc fragment)
- **opsonisation** (improving the efficiency of phagocytic uptake via the Fc fragment)
- **prevention of adherence** (through binding to micro-organism adherins)
- **neutralisation of toxins**
- **antibody-dependent cell cytotoxicity** (through natural killer cell recognition of bound antibody via the Fc fragment).

T lymphocytes are important for the overall control of the immune response and for the recognition and killing of infected host cells. In contrast to B lymphocytes, they can only respond to antigens presented on cell surfaces and not free antigen:

- Every nucleated cell expresses a sample of its cytosolic molecules on the cell surface in association with **Class I HLA** molecules; if the cell is manufacturing 'foreign' antigens, such as will occur in intracellular infections, particularly viral, this will be detected by **cytotoxic** T cells and they will kill the infected cell (**Fig. 12.5**).
- Phagocytic cells express a sample of breakdown products from engulfed material, particularly non-viral pathogens, on their surface in association with **Class II HLA** molecules, a set of molecules largely restricted to antigen-presenting cells. Foreign antigens will be recognised by **helper** T cells, whose post-activation effector cells (Th1, Th0 or Th2) produce a range of cytokines that will determine the nature of the subsequent immune response (**Figs 12.1 and 12.5**).

There is considerable movement of immune cells throughout the body:

- T cells mature in the thymus and B cells in the bone marrow (**primary lymphoid organs**) in the fetus, before moving to **secondary lymphoid organs** such as the spleen, lymph nodes and mucosa-associated lymphoid tissue (**MALT**).
- Phagocytes and debris pass from the site of infection to the secondary lymphoid organs, where lymphocyte stimulation takes place. The activated lymphocytes, and other inflammatory cells such as platelets and monocytes, are then directed back to the site of infection by activated complement factors and chemo-attractants, released by leucocytes and damaged cells at the site.

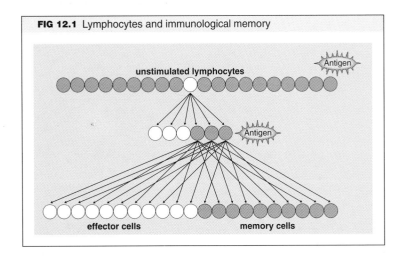

FIG 12.1 Lymphocytes and immunological memory

unstimulated lymphocytes

Antigen

Antigen

effector cells   memory cells

TABLE 12.1

Immunoglobulins and their functions

Isotype	Configuration	Complement fixation	Cells that react with Fc receptors	Serum concentration
IgM	Pentamer	Good	Lymphocytes	Moderate
IgG$_1$	Monomer	Good	Widespread	Most abundant
IgG$_2$	Monomer	Poor	Lymphocytes, platelets	Abundant
IgG$_3$	Monomer	Good	Widespread	Moderate
IgG$_4$	Monomer	Absent	Neutrophils, lymphocytes, platelets	Moderate
IgA$_1$	Monomer	Absent	None	Moderate
IgA$_2$	Dimer	Absent	None	Little (present in mucosal secretions)
IgD	Monomer	Absent	None	Very little
IgE	Monomer	Absent	Mast cells, eosinophils, lymphocytes	Very little (attached to mast cells)

FIG 12.2 The lymphocyte family

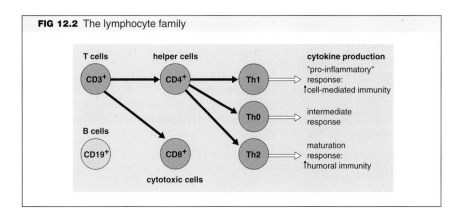

FIG 12.3 Basic structure of an antibody molecule

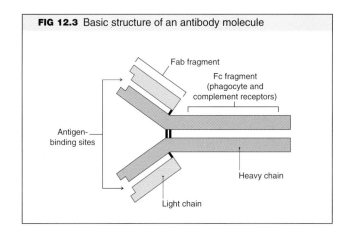

FIG 12.4 Antibody production during infection

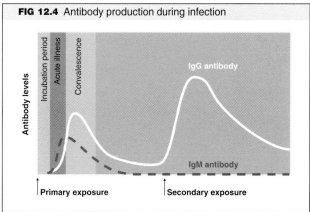

FIG 12.5 T cell recognition of antigen

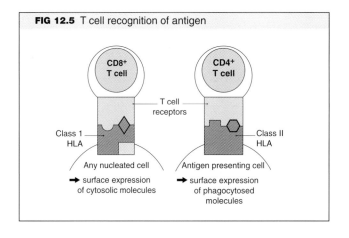

27

SAQ 2 — Immunity to infection

Questions

1. Define the following terms: antigen, immunogen, epitope, hapten.

2. Name three infections that are more severe in patients with selective immunoglobulin deficiency.

3. List three infections which are associated with deficiency of specific components of complement.

4. Describe the mechanism by which viruses evade the immune response.

5. Outline the specific immune response to protozoa and helminths (parasites).

6. What cells are involved in phagocytosis of microbes?

7. What are defensins?

8. Draw a simple diagram of the phagocytosis and intracellular digestion of a microbe by a neutrophil.

9. Give three examples of microbes that interfere with phagocytic function.

10. Cite examples of a virus, a bacterium, a fungus and a protozoon that can replicate in macrophages.

Answers

1. An **antigen** is a substance capable of causing an immune response, i.e. it can elicit antibody and interact specifically with that antibody. An **immunogen** is a term used to describe a substance that has the first of those properties. A **hapten** is a substance that is not immunogenic by itself but in combination can react specifically with antibody. An **epitope** or antigenic determinant is that part of an antigen that is recognised by elicited antibodies.

2. Specific immunoglobulin deficiency is usually congenital, e.g. infantile X-linked agammaglobulinaemia. In such children recurrent infections with pyogenic bacteria occur after the disappearance of maternal antibody. Such infections include causes of pneumonia, such as the Pneumococcus and *Haemophilus influenzae*. In contrast, they handle most viral infections with the exception of enteroviruses.

3. Specific complement deficiencies are rare inherited conditions, although low general complement activity is a 'normal' feature in the fetus which predisposes the premature infant to infection, particularly with capsulate bacteria. Examples of specific complement deficiency and the predisposed infections are:

Complement deficiency	Infections
• C2	Pneumococcal septicaemia
• C6–C9	Meningococcal and gonococcal infection.

4. Viruses evade the immune response by two main mechanisms:

   • Antigenic variation. Viruses, especially those with RNA genomes, evolve rapidly, and viable mutants can arise with each replicative cycle. Significant antigenic variation is responsible for the lack of long-term efficacy of influenza vaccination.
   • Viruses can also suppress the immune system. This may be by direct destruction of immune cells as occurs in HIV or by subtler mechanisms. EBV has a gene that is homologous to the mammalian IL-10 gene; this may possibly reduce macrophage function and the release of cytokines required for an antiviral, Th1, response, such as IL-1, TNF and IL-12.

5. Parasite infections tend to be chronic, implying a weak immune response, but are kept in check by:

   • specific IgE and eosinophilia — hallmarks of a Th2 type response
   • granuloma formation to wall off the infection
   • cytokines and CD4+ T helper cells, involved in resistance to Leishmania infection
   • specific cytotoxic T lymphocytes (CTLs) induced by protozoa, such as malaria, that replicate inside cells.

6. Epithelial cells can be phagocytic, but it is the professional phagocyte that is most important in infections: macrophages and polymorphonuclear cells (neutrophils, basophils and eosinophils).

7. **Defensins** are cationic peptides of about 30 amino acids produced by neutrophils and macrophages with antibiotic-like activity. They are active against a wide range of microbes, including *S. aureus, E. coli, P. aeruginosa* and herpes simplex.

8. See Figure, p. 121.

9. Many bacteria, such as *H. influenzae* and *S. pneumoniae*, produce an external capsule that resists take-up by the phagocyte. Others such as *P. aeruginosa* produce an exotoxin that kills phagocytic cells. Mycobacteria are taken up within cells but prevent lysosomal fusion and therefore digestion.

10. Several micro-organisms can replicate within macrophages:

Type of micro-organism	Examples
• virus	measles poxviruses
• bacteria	*Rickettsia* spp. mycobacteria *Listeria monocytogenes* *Legionella pneumophila* *Brucella* spp.
• fungi	*Cryptococcus neoformans*
• protozoa	*Toxoplasma* spp. *Leishmania* spp. *Trypanosoma* spp.

13 Diagnosis of infectious disease

Timely and accurate diagnosis of infectious disease requires clinical acumen and liaison between clinician and microbiologist. As in all clinical diagnoses, the starting point must be a clear **history** and full **examination**. Particular points to establish in the history are:

- timing and nature of fevers (constant, nightly, rigors, sweats)
- contact with other cases of infection
- predisposing factors (diabetes, immunosuppression, chronic obstructive airways disease, etc.)
- history of recent or recurrent infection (urinary tract, skin, etc.)
- travel history and relevant immunisations/prophylaxis
- animal contacts
- recent or current antimicrobial therapy
- drug allergies.

Some patients have symptoms that clearly indicate the focus of infection; others have fever without localising features. Systemic infections may present with potentially misleading symptoms (e.g. cough in typhoid and diarrhoea in Legionnaires' disease). The examination should include:

- the temperature (noting the site where this was taken)
- a search for local or generalised lymphadenopathy
- the skin (signs of breaks in the skin — trauma, ulcers, wounds, i.v. line sites and description of rashes)
- careful examination of each organ system, particularly the respiratory and gastrointestinal tracts.

A review of the clinical features may establish a diagnosis without specific investigations. This is typically the case in general practice in mild upper respiratory tract infections where the majority of cases are viral in origin and treatment is largely symptomatic and unlikely to be influenced by cultures or serology. In other cases (e.g. otitis media without perforation) suitable specimens may not be readily accessible and treatment is usually empirical. Many general practitioners (GPs) treat uncomplicated urinary tract infections without sending urine for culture. However, the choice of empirical antimicrobial treatment must be based on up-to-date **susceptibility data** from local isolates. Similarly, even in conditions that are usually self-limiting (e.g. influenza and infectious diarrhoea), **epidemiological data** from specimens is essential for effective **communicable disease control** (e.g. vaccine development and food safety measures).

In more severe disease the clinical findings direct the choice of primary **investigations**. Of particular value is the **total and differential white cell count**. Basic biochemical investigations such as urea, creatinine, electrolytes and liver function tests give an indication of the severity of disease and renal or hepatic impairment. Conventional **imaging techniques** such as X-rays are now frequently supplemented by scans using ultrasound, tomography and magnetic resonance and direct visualisation using endoscopic devices.

Appropriate cultures must always be collected before antimicrobial therapy is started. An important exception to this rule is suspected meningococcal infection where GPs are advised to give parenteral penicillin immediately. First consideration should be given to **blood cultures**. Although the positivity rate is low (typically around 10% in the UK), positive cultures are extremely helpful in both diagnosis and treatment. As with all specimens from normally sterile sites, care must be taken to avoid contamination. Clinical features will guide the collection of other appropriate specimens from specific sites. The general principles of specimen collection are given in **Table 13.1**.

Organism detection in specimens may involve a variety of methods (**Table 13.2**). Many of these techniques are rapid and provide presumptive diagnoses within minutes of specimen receipt. **Culture** is still the commonest detection technique — it is cheap and provides isolates for susceptibility tests but is slow and labour intensive.

Sophisticated **molecular techniques** are increasingly available and invaluable for organisms that are difficult, slow or impossible to culture. It is also possible to detect the molecular basis of resistance (e.g. rifampicin resistance in *M. tuberculosis*), and this may have more widespread application in the future.

Infectious agents may also be detected by **serological techniques** — the antibody response (**Table 13.3**). Antibody production may not be detectable at the time of presentation, and specimens are classically collected as paired acute and convalescent sera. A four-fold rise in titre confirms a significant response in acute infections. A single raised titre is suggestive of infection but may be diagnostic in chronic infections (e.g. HBV, HIV). Assays that detect specific IgM are also available for many infections.

Skin tests have a limited role in diagnosis but the Mantoux (tuberculin) test is still widely used to demonstrate cell-mediated hypersensitivity to *M. tuberculosis*.

TABLE 13.1

Collection of specimens

Aspect	Measures to be taken
Container	Have appropriate container available before collecting specimen
Site	Ensure correct site sampled, e.g. throat (versus mouth), cervix (versus vagina)
Quality	Avoid contamination from adjacent sites — skin, mouth, genital tract, etc.
Quantity	Collect adequate volume — pus is preferable to swab
Transport	Use appropriate transport media for swabs (bacterial, viral) Ensure specimen containers are tightly sealed Ensure specimen transported rapidly to laboratory or held at appropriate temperature
Labelling	Specimen must be clearly labelled with patient's name, the site and date of sample
Request form	Complete fully — sender, patient, clinical details (including antimicrobial therapy), specimen (including date & time)
High risk	Specimens from patients with known or suspected high-risk pathogens must be marked and transported in a sealed bag

TABLE 13.2

Detection of organisms

Time scale	Method	Examples
Minutes or hours	Direct microscopy	Urines (cells, organisms) Dark-ground microscopy (spirochaetes) Electron microscopy (viruses)
	Staining	Gram film (bacteria and fungi) Ziehl–Neelsen (mycobacteria) Lactophenol cotton blue (fungi) Iodine (protozoa)
	Antigen detection: 1. agglutination	Pneumococci, meningococci cryptococci, candida
	2. fluoresence	Chlamydia, RSV
	3. ELISA	Hepatitis B, rotavirus
	Products of metabolism	Gas liquid chromatography (fatty acid products of anaerobes)
	Nucleic acid probes	PCR (HIV, Hepatitis C, *M. tuberculosis*) LCR (chlamydia)
One or more days	Solid & liquid culture	Most bacteria, yeasts,
	Tissue culture	Some viruses (e.g. Herpes simplex)
	Toxin detection	*Cl. difficile* cytotoxin in cell culture
Weeks	Lowenstein–Jensen agar	Mycobacteria
	Tissue culture	Slower-growing viruses (e.g. CMV)

TABLE 13.3

Serological techniques

Method	Examples
Agglutination	Legionnaires' disease (microagglutination test)
Haemagglutination	Paul–Bunnell test (infectious mononucleosis)
Haemagglutination inhibition	Influenza
Neutralisation	Anti-streptolysin O test (ASOT)
Precipitation	Aspergillus
Complement fixation	Mycoplasma, psittacosis, Q fever
Fluorescence	Legionnaires' disease Syphilis — fluorescent treponemal antibody test (FTA)
ELISA	Syphilis

Diseases caused by micro-organisms

14 Upper respiratory tract infections

The upper respiratory tract (**Fig. 14.1**) is the initial site of infection or a site of colonisation for most infections of the respiratory tract. It is also the site for a number of resident organisms, the prevalence of which will vary in individuals (**Table 14.1**). Some of these resident flora have the propensity to be pathogenic. Infections of the upper respiratory tract (URTIs) are the commonest acute illness.

Common colds / rhinitis Children suffer 2–6 colds per year in industrialised countries, with this frequency halving in adulthood. This high incidence of colds is attributable to the high number of viruses and serotypes involved. Both aerosol and fomite transmission contribute to spread of infection.

The principal findings of rhinorrhoea and sneezing are found in almost all cases. In addition there may be sore throat, headaches and constitutional upset with fever. Earache is frequent in childhood. The diagnosis of the syndrome is clinical; laboratory identification is not required because of the current absence of appropriate antiviral therapy. Anti-rhinoviral therapy is, however, a possibility as drugs are developed that block the interaction between the major host cell receptor (ICAM-1) and the virus anti-receptor in a canyon that occurs on the surface of the viral capsid. Symptomatic therapy with analgesics and decongestants is commonly employed. Vaccine development is hindered by the diverse aetiology.

Influenza Unlike common colds, which are non-life-threatening illnesses, much mortality is attributable to influenza, particularly in the elderly and those with underlying cardiopulmonary disease. Clinically, there are three features that distinguish influenza infection from common colds: an acute onset, presence of a fever in almost all cases (occurs in the minority of common colds) and more marked constitutional upset with myalgia. Amantadine and rimantadine are used in the treatment and prophylaxis of influenza A infections. A vaccine is recommended for patients with underlying chronic cardiopulmonary disease, chronic renal failure, or diabetes mellitus, and in the immunosuppressed. This vaccine is changed annually because the virus undergoes genetic change either through minor sequence changes (resulting in '**antigenic drift**') or through recombination (resulting in '**antigenic shift**') which produce changes in one or both surface proteins, the haemagglutin (H) or neuraminidase (N). Antigenic shift increases the likelihood of a widespread pandemic, as even partial prior immunity to a completely new strain is absent.

Sore throat / pharyngitis and tonsillitis Over two-thirds of sore throats are viral in aetiology and may be a continuum of infection of the nasal mucosa (common cold). *Streptococcus pyogenes* is the commonest bacterial cause and can be associated with severe complications (**Table 14.2**).

Diphtheria is caused by *Corynebacterium diphtheriae*. There is much local inflammation of the nasopharynx, with a characteristic 'bull neck' appearance from enlarged lymph nodes. Toxigenic strains of *C. diphtheriae* produce a polypeptide that causes local destruction of epithelial cells and spreads systemically to cause myocarditis and polyneuritis.

The aetiological diagnosis is made by culture of a throat swab or by serological assays. With diphtheria, toxin production should also be sought. Most viral sore throats are self-limiting and are managed symptomatically. *S. pyogenes* infections should be treated (most frequently with a penicillin) to prevent complications. Diphtheria toxin can be neutralised with antitoxin. Contacts of diphtheria should be screened and given booster vaccination and/or chemoprophylaxis as appropriate.

Sinusitis / acute otitis media These conditions are most frequently a complication of common colds but may also be due to secondary bacterial invaders (**Fig. 14.1**). Localised pain is the most frequent symptom, but children with otitis media may present with unexplained fever or vomiting. If chronic infection results, surgery may be necessary in addition to antibiotics.

Epiglottitis This is most commonly a disease of young children as a result of spread of bacteria from the nasopharynx. *Haemophilus influenzae* type b is the classic cause, but other bacteria may now be more frequent. Bacteraemia is frequent, and epiglottitis may present as an acute medical emergency with respiratory obstruction. Antibiotics may need to be given intravenously.

Tracheitis / laryngotracheitis This causes hoarseness and retrosternal discomfort on both inspiration and expiration. Parainfluenza (and other) viruses cause swelling of the mucous membrane that results in inspiratory stridor, termed 'croup'. Diagnosis of the specific aetiology is made by identification from a throat swab or serologically.

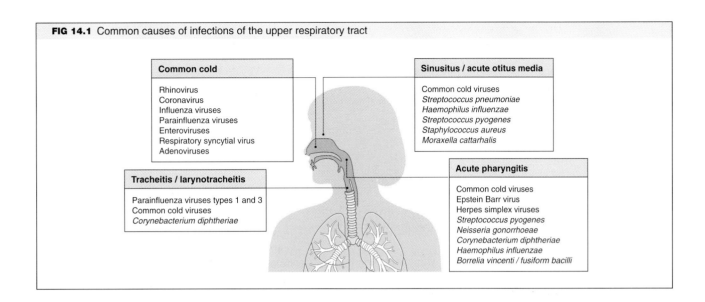

FIG 14.1 Common causes of infections of the upper respiratory tract

Common cold

Rhinovirus
Coronavirus
Influenza viruses
Parainfluenza viruses
Enteroviruses
Respiratory syncytial virus
Adenoviruses

Sinusitus / acute otitus media

Common cold viruses
Streptococcus pneumoniae
Haemophilus influenzae
Streptococcus pyogenes
Staphylococcus aureus
Moraxella cattarhalis

Tracheitis / larynotracheitis

Parainfluenza viruses types 1 and 3
Common cold viruses
Corynebacterium diphtheriae

Acute pharyngitis

Common cold viruses
Epstein Barr virus
Herpes simplex viruses
Streptococcus pyogenes
Neisseria gonorrhoeae
Corynebacterium diphtheriae
Haemophilus influenzae
Borrelia vincenti / fusiform bacilli

TABLE 14.1

Normal flora of the upper respiratory tract

Common (> 50%)
- *Streptococcus mutans* and other alpha-haemolytic streptococci
- *Neisseria* spp.
- corynebacteria
- *Bacteroides* spp.
- *Veillonella* spp.
- other anaerobic cocci
- fusiform bacteria
- *Candida albicans*
- *Haemophilus influenzae*
- *Entamoeba gingivalis*

Less common (< 50%)
- *Streptococcus pyogenes*
- *Streptococcus pneumoniae*
- *Neisseria meningitidis*
- *Staphylococcus aureus*
- others

TABLE 14.2

Complications of *Streptococcus pyogenes* infection

- peritonsillar abscess ('quinsy')
- scarlet fever, a punctate erythematous rash resulting from those strains that produce a vasodilatory toxin
- rheumatic fever, which is caused by an autoimmune response to bacterial cell wall that damages heart (myocarditis or pericarditis), joints (polyarthritis) and occasionally nervous system ('Sydenham's' chorea)
- rheumatic carditis from damage to heart valves
- acute glomerulonephritis from immune complex deposition in the
- glomeruli.

Lower respiratory tract infections

15

The lower respiratory tract is defined as below and including the larynx. Due to the **mucociliary escalator**, the complex and abundant bacterial flora of the upper tract is much reduced in the larynx and trachea, and the bronchi are sterile in health. Respiratory tract infections are the most frequent cause of GP consultation. The great majority of infections are, however, self-limiting, and a provisional diagnosis should be based upon the signs and symptoms (**Fig. 15.1**), with laboratory investigation confined to those that may be serious (**Table 15.1**). Different organisms characteristically affect different parts of the respiratory tract, although, once infection has been initiated, the inflammation can become widespread.

Airway infection Although infection in the larynx and/or trachea and/or the bronchi may occur at any age, it is extremely common in the young (**croup**) and in elderly smokers.

- The diagnosis of *Bordetella pertussis* infection should be made clinically on the basis of the characteristic severe paroxysmal spasmodic 'whooping' cough, as laboratory confirmation is slow and unreliable. Erythromycin may reduce spread, but it is rarely possible to give the antibiotic sufficiently early for this to be worthwhile; vaccination is more helpful.
- Influenza may be complicated by super-infection with bacteria, especially pneumococcal and staphylococcal pneumonia. Influenza vaccine should be given to all 'at risk' persons in the autumn, and the drug amantidine may be useful if given early in infection.
- RSV causes a severe bronchiolitis in those aged less than 2 (and the elderly), which may either be fatal or produce sufficient lung damage to bring about asthma later in life. It is easily transmitted within hospitals but may respond to the drug ribavirin.

Parenchymal infection (pneumonia) Pneumonia is infection involving the lung interstitium manifest as fever, increased respiratory difficulty and cough productive of purulent sputum. It is most commonly caused by a bacterium in adults, detectable by culture of sputum (not saliva).

In contrast to **bronchopneumonia**, in **atypical pneumonia** there is less production of sputum, but the systemic symptoms and chest X-ray changes are greater than might be suspected given the few signs on chest examination. The severity of pneumonia and likely outcome can be judged by simple measures such as respiratory rate, blood pressure, blood urea, O_2 saturation and pulse rate. *Mycoplasma* and *Chlamydia* (causes of atypical pneumonia) can infect the previously healthy, as can *S. pneumoniae*, which is the only cause of a pneumonia with a truly **lobar** distribution. The remaining causes of bronchopneumonia are more likely to infect those in poor health and to be responsible for acute exacerbation of Chronic Obstructive Pulmonary Disease (COPD), although most exacerbations are due to viral causes. *L. pneumophila* is spread by aerosol, such as those created by poorly-maintained showers and air-conditioners, and typically affects the borderline immunocompromised — for example, heavy-drinking, heavy-smoking elderly persons returning from a holiday in the sun!

The choice of antibiotic for a community-acquired pneumonia is described in **Fig. 15.2**; a hospital-acquired pneumonia is more likely to be caused by antibiotic-resistant organisms, and a second or third generation cephalosporin may be the treatment of choice.

Tuberculosis This was a decreasing problem until recently when the numbers started to rise again, particularly amongst the poor, immigrant groups and HIV-positive patients. However, it should never be forgotten as a cause of serious disease. The chest is usually the main site of infection, classically causing cough, haemoptysis, pleuritic pain, weight loss and night sweats, but it may disseminate to any site in the body. Antibiotic resistance may arise during treatment, which usually involves prolonged therapy with pyrazinamide, isoniazid, ethambutol and rifampicin.

Cystic fibrosis In cystic fibrosis, the combination of thickened secretions and repeated viral, *S. aureus* and *H. influenzae* infections in early life lead to severe bronchiectasis; chronic infection with *Pseudomonas aeruginosa*, and sometimes *Burkholderia cepacia*, results in fatal destruction of the lung in spite of frequent courses of potent i.v. and nebulised antibiotics. However, the life expectancy has increased dramatically with improved management and may do so further with gene therapy.

TABLE 15.1

Diagnosis of lower respiratory tract infection

	Sample	Test	Infectious agent
Laryngo-tracheo-bronchitis	Pernasal swab	Antigen detection & bacterial culture	*B. pertussis*
	Nasopharyngeal aspirate	Antigen detection & viral culture	Influenza
	Acute & convalescent sera	Antibody levels	Influenza
Bronchiolitis	Nasopharyngeal aspirate	Antigen detection & viral culture	Respiratory syncitial virus (RSV)
Pneumonia	Sputum	Bacterial culture	All causes of bronchopneumonia & *L. pneumophila*
		Antigen detection	*S. pneumoniae* & *L. pneumophila*
	Urine	Antigen detection	*S. pneumoniae* & *L. pneumophila*
	Acute & convalescent sera	Antibody levels	All causes of viral & atypical pneumonia
Tuberculosis	Sputum	Ziehl–Neelsen stain & mycobacterial culture	*M. tuberculosis* & atypical mycobacteria

FIG 15.1 Aetiology and symptoms of lower respiratory tract infection

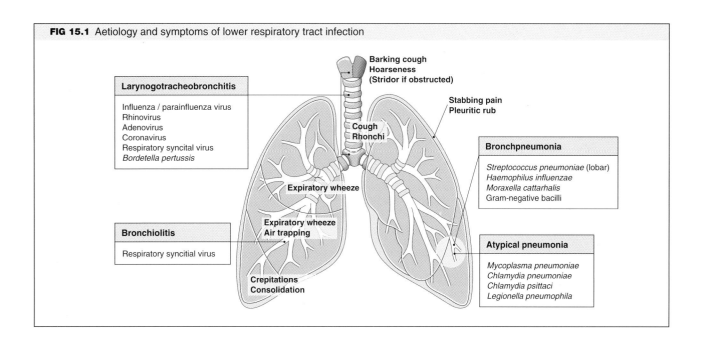

FIG 15.2 Antibiotics for use in community-acquired pneumonia

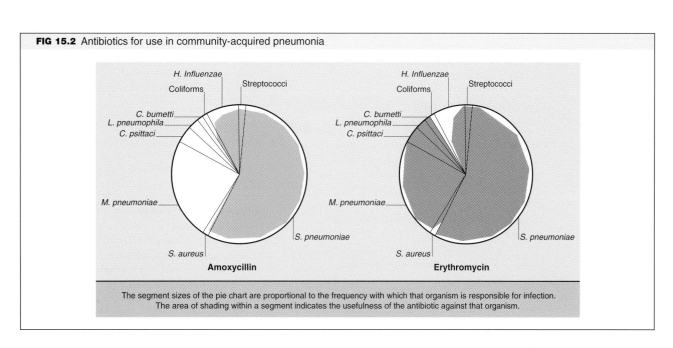

The segment sizes of the pie chart are proportional to the frequency with which that organism is responsible for infection. The area of shading within a segment indicates the usefulness of the antibiotic against that organism.

16 Meningitis

Infection of the meninges follows invasion of pathogens across the **blood–brain** or **blood–cerebrospinal fluid barrier**. In rare instances organisms may gain direct access following surgery, trauma or (in amoebic infections) directly through the cribriform plate. The characteristic clinical features of meningitis are:

- headache
- irritability or drowsiness, sometimes with alteration of consciousness
- fever
- neck stiffness
- photophobia
- Positive Kernig's sign (pain in the lumbar region on straight-leg raising).

Most infections are acute and the commonest pathogens are viruses, especially in children and young adults. Patients with **viral meningitis** often present with a history of an influenza-like illness with headache, sore throat and muscle pains. The features of meningitis then follow but tend to be milder than in bacterial infections and less rapid in onset. The viral causes of meningitis are shown in **Table 16.1**. Most cases of viral meningitis resolve completely without specific treatment.

Mumps virus is second to enteroviruses as a cause of meningitis. The most prominent manifestation is, however, parotitis. Epididymo-orchitis may, uncommonly, result in sterility; thyroiditis and pancreatitis, meningo-encephalitis, myocarditis and arthritis are rare complications.

In contrast, bacterial meningitis may be life-threatening and have serious sequelae for those who survive (**Table 16.2**). Whilst it may be impossible to predict the causative agent from the clinical features, some pathogens are commoner at certain ages.

Bacterial meningitis

Neonatal meningitis may be classified as **early-** (within 7 days of birth) or **late-onset disease** (occurring between 1 week and 3 months). Early infections are acquired from the mother, whereas late infections may result from cross-infection after birth. The commonest causes of early-onset disease are Group B β-haemolytic streptococci and coliforms such as *Escherichia coli*. *Listeria monocytogenes* is less common but, like Group B β-haemolytic streptococci, may also cause late-onset disease.

The majority of cases of bacterial meningitis occur in childhood. The introduction of Hib vaccine against type b strains of *Haemophilus influenzae* has significantly reduced the incidence of invasive infections caused by this organism. The commonest cause is now *Neisseria meningitidis*. The three common serotypes A, B and C vary in prevalence around the world, but B and C are commonest in western Europe. Acute meningococcal disease may present as a septicaemic illness without meningitis. Such infections are often characterised by a petechial rash, and patients may develop endotoxic shock. Research into the mediators of meningococcal toxaemia has lead to searches for novel therapeutic interventions in addition to antibiotic therapy. Meningitis caused by *Streptococcus pneumoniae* occurs at all ages but particularly in children under 2 years, the elderly and those with immune defects (e.g. sickle-cell disease and post-splenectomy).

Meningitis in adolescents and young adults is most commonly caused by meningococci. In later life, pneumococci are more likely pathogens. *Listeria monocytogenes* is a relatively rare cause but should be considered particularly in pregnant and immunocompromised patients.

Tuberculous meningitis Tubercle bacilli may spread from distant sites via the lymphatic system and the bloodstream, particularly in acute miliary tuberculosis. The onset of disease is often gradual with days or weeks of general malaise before the onset of meningeal features. Diagnosis may be difficult in the early stages, but localising neurological signs such as cranial nerve palsies are helpful.

Diagnosis Blood cultures should always be taken, preferably before antibiotics are started. Although there are contra-indications (especially raised intracranial pressure) to lumbar puncture, examination of cerebrospinal fluid is advisable whenever possible. CSF findings are shown in **Table 16.3**. Additional investigations in suspected meningococcal disease should include the following, particularly if the patient has already received antibiotics:

- throat swab
- acute serum for meningococcal antibodies and antigen detection
- blood for meningococcal polymerase chain reaction (PCR)
- scrapings of petechiae for Gram stain and culture.

Treatment and prophylaxis of bacterial meningitis Treatment must be prompt, and immediate parenteral penicillin (before hospital admission) is recommended in suspected meningococcal disease. Appropriate antimicrobials are shown in **Table 16.2**. Chemoprophylaxis of close contacts is recommended in meningococcal (and Hib) disease to reduce the risk of secondary cases. In addition, contacts of cases of serotypes A and C meningococcal disease may be vaccinated — a reliable type B vaccine is still awaited. Patients over 2 years of age at increased risk of pneumococcal disease should be immunised with a polyvalent vaccine.

TABLE 16.1

Viral causes of meningitis

Virus family	Virus
Picornavirus	Echo
	Coxsackie
	Polio
Paramyxovirus	Mumps
Herpesvirus	Herpes simplex
	Varicella zoster
	Epstein–Barr
Arenavirus	Lymphocytic choriomeningitis
Togavirus	Louping ill
	Japanese encephalitis
	E & W equine encephalitis
Retrovirus	HIV

TABLE 16.2

Bacterial causes of meningitis

Bacteria	Typical patients[a]	Treatment[b]
Neisseria meningitidis	Children and teenagers	Penicillin
Strep. pneumoniae	< 2 years and elderly	Penicillin, ceftriaxone
Haemophilus influenzae	Unvaccinated children > 5 years	Ceftriaxone
Group B streptococci Coliforms (e.g. *E. coli*) *Listeria monocytogenes*	Neonates	Penicillin & gentamicin
Mycobacterium tuberculosis	Young & middle-aged More common in non-Caucasians	Isoniazid, rifampicin, pyrazinamide
Coagulase-negative staphylococci	CSF shunt in situ	Shunt removal or intrathecal antibiotics
Staph. aureus	Post-neurosurgery	Flucloxacillin or cephalosporin

[a]Infections are not restricted to these groups
[b]Specific treatment depends on susceptibilities of the isolate

TABLE 16.3

CSF findings in meningitis

	Pressure	Cells/μL	Predominant cell type	Glucose[a] (mmol/L)	Protein (g/L)
Normal	100–200 mmHg	0–5	Lymphocytes	2.8–4.4	0.15–0.45
Acute bacterial meningitis	↑	200–10 000	Neutrophils	↓↓	0.5–3.0
Viral meningitis	N or ↑	100–1000	Lymphocytes	N	0.5–1.0
Tuberculous meningitis	N or ↑	50–500	Lymphocytes	↓	1–6

[a]The ratio of CSF/blood glucose is more important that the absolute level — normal CSF glucose is approximately 60% of blood glucose

Case study 1

A 22 year old sociology student feels mildly unwell over the weekend and thinks that she may be coming down with a cold. However, she rallied sufficiently to go out drinking on Sunday night (5 pints of lager in the Semantics & Firkin) followed by a fish supper and a pickled egg. The next morning she feels much worse than she usually does on a Monday — she is drowsy, feels hot and has a headache (particularly when the curtains are opened).

Questions

1. What is your differential diagnosis?

2. If you were the GP called to see her, what must you particularly look for in your examination?

3. She has three small reddish-purple non-blanching patches on her back and has a positive Kernig's sign. What is your diagnosis and what are you going to do about it?

4. You are the house officer and this is your first suspected case of meningococcal meningitis. How would you investigate this patient to confirm your diagnosis?

5. Analysis of the CSF is as shown below. Does this confirm or exclude a diagnosis of meningococcal infection?

   - red cell count — 50×10^6 cells/μL (normal ≈ 0)
   - white cell count
     — 1250×10^6 cells/μL (normal ≤ 5)
     — 90% polymorphs
     — 10% lymphocytes
   - protein — 0.8 g/L (normal range 0.15–0.45 g/L)
   - glucose
     — CSF 1.2 mmol/L (normal range CSF glucose $\geq 60\%$ serum glucose)
     — serum 5.8 mmol/L
   - no organisms seen by Gram stain and microscopy.

6. What antibiotics would you choose to treat this woman — justify your choice!

7. Do you need to inform anybody about this case — explain your answer.

8. What immunological deficit would you look for in a patient with repeated episodes of meningococcal infection?

Answers

1. A 'hangover', respiratory tract infection or meningitis (viral or bacterial) might all be considered.

2. Meningitis is the most serious of these conditions; whilst you might examine her chest, for example, you must look for neck stiffness and a petechial rash.

3. Meningococcal septicaemia and meningitis; give benzylpenicillin (e.g. 1.2 g i.m. or i.v.) immediately and arrange for urgent hospital admission.

4. The full work-up might include:

   • lumbar puncture (if no evidence of raised intracranial pressure), the sample to be sent for both bacteriological and virological analysis

   • blood for bacteriological culture (2–3 sets if possible)

   • clotted blood sample for antigen detection/serology (a follow-up sample will also be required if the diagnosis is not established by the time of convalescence)

   • an EDTA blood sample for PCR

   • skin scrape or punch biopsy of the petechial rash for microscopy/bacterial culture

   • a throat swab for bacterial and viral culture

   • faeces for viral culture.

5. This is typical of a bacterial meningitis and would be extremely unlikely to be found in viral meningitis. The use of antibiotics by the GP may explain why there are no bacteria visible on microscopy, and it is still most likely to be a case of meningococcal infection on clinical grounds.

6. Benzyl penicillin is the treatment of choice as it is cheap, narrow spectrum and effective. A third-generation cephalosporin is an alternative which is equally effective although not strictly necessary unless this is one of the very rare meningococcal isolates that is penicillin-insensitive.

7. The Consultant in Communicable Disease Control (Consultant in Public Health Medicine in Scotland) should be informed. This is to allow the tracing of close contacts of this case and attempt the eradication of meningococcal carriage from them and so prevent further spread (using rifampicin, ciprofloxacin or ceftriaxone) and also give vaccine prophylaxis if it is serogroup C (or A) disease.

8. The most important would be a complement deficiency: C3 deficiency may lead to severe disseminated infection with capsulate bacteria such as *N. meningitidis* and *S. pneumoniae*; deficiency in C5, C6, C7 or C8 tends to give rather more benign episodes of recurrent meningococcal bacteraemia. Meningitis may also be the first sign of an abnormal communication between the CSF and the nasal passages.

17 Encephalitis and other nervous system infections

Infections occur in the brain (**encephalitis** and **brain abscess**), spinal cord (**myelitis**), nerves (**neuritis** or **polyneuritis**), or a combination of these. The nervous system is normally sterile, and infections have to traverse either the blood–brain barrier or be directly inoculated (**Fig. 17.1**). Unlike meningitis, which often recovers without sequelae, nervous tissue has poor repair mechanisms, and tissue damage leads to long-term sequelae.

Encephalitis / brain abscess Encephalitis is predominantly a viral disease (**Table 17.1**) with herpes simplex infection being the most common in the UK. Cerebral dysfunction presents as behavioural disturbance, fits and diminished consciousness. If progressive, then localised neurological signs, coma and death may occur. Diagnosis of the condition is clinical with confirmation from imaging and electroencephalography (EEG). Virus may also be detectable in the cerebrospinal fluid (CSF) but may not be cultivable. Brain biopsy offers the definitive means of diagnosis but is only used in specialist centres. HSV encephalitis has a 70% mortality unless treated with aciclovir. Rabies is fatal but can be treated with post-exposure prophylaxis, as the long incubation period allows time for an adequate immune response.

By contrast, **brain abscesses** are predominantly bacterial in origin and arise because of spread from other sites such as infected cardiac valves and bones, mastoid sinuses and chronic middle ear infection; pathogens include *S. aureus*, streptococci, Gram-negative bacilli, anaerobes and are often mixed. Localised neurological signs are common. Multiple abscesses/cysts may be due to either bacteria or *Echinococcus granulosus* (termed hydatid disease), *Toxocara* spp. (toxocariasis) or tapeworm infection (cysticercosis), which are zoonoses. Diagnosis is by imaging and, for the helminth diseases, by serology. Single abscesses are treated empirically with antibiotics such as ceftriaxone and metronidazole, usually in conjunction with surgical drainage. Appropriate chemotherapy is used for helminth infections, with consideration of poor transfer of most antimicrobials across the non-inflamed blood–brain barrier.

Myelitis This may accompany encephalitis (**encephalomyelitis**) but may present as the predominant feature. **Poliomyelitis** is an infection of the anterior horn cells and motor neurones with poliovirus, and other enteroviruses, causing a flaccid paralysis which may lead to residual muscle wasting from disuse; paralytic poliomyelitis occurs, however, in fewer than 1% of poliovirus infections. **Rabies** may cause an ascending flaccid paralysis if bites occur on the lower extremities.

Transverse myelitis with bilateral flaccid or spastic paraparesis now occurs more commonly with other infectious agents as poliovirus vaccination is implemented word-wide (**Table 17.2**).

Neuritis / polyneuritis Direct infection of nerves with Schwann cell degeneration, which may be followed by axonal degeneration, results from infections with *Mycobacterium leprae, Trypanosoma* spp., *Microsporidia* spp. and cytomegalovirus (CMV). Flaccid paralysis results. Varicella-zoster virus causes the Ramsay-Hunt syndrome, which presents with vesicles in the ear canal and a unilateral facial nerve palsy.

Infections such as tetanus, botulism and diphtheria produce **neurotoxins** which interfere with synaptic transmission.

Guillain–Barré syndrome is an ascending bilateral paralysis which is generally preceded by an infection up to 4 weeks prior to onset. Campylobacter gastroenteritis is the commonest precipitant, but other gastrointestinal and respiratory tract infective causes have also been noted. An autoimmune aetiology is postulated.

Bell's palsy, a normally transient unilateral facial palsy, may be aetiologically associated with herpes simplex infection, although there is little benefit from the use of aciclovir.

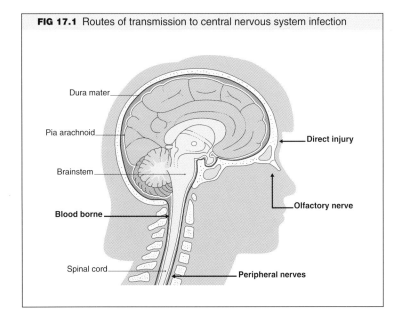

FIG 17.1 Routes of transmission to central nervous system infection

Dura mater

Pia arachnoid

Brainstem

Blood borne

Spinal cord

Direct injury

Olfactory nerve

Peripheral nerves

TABLE 17.1

Causes of encephalitis

Cause	Features
Herpes simplex virus (HSV)	Bitemporal localisation detectable on CT, MRI & EEG. HSV-2 common in neonates, HSV-1 in adults
Mumps virus	Meningoencephalitis may precede parotitis
Eastern & Western equine, St Louis, California encephalitis viruses (Toga/Bunyaviruses)	Mosquito-borne. Found in parts of N. America
Rabies virus (Rhabdovirus)	Transmitted by bites from dogs, foxes, bats & other mammals. Incubation period of weeks to months. Fatal if not treated
Tick-borne encephalitis virus(es) — (Flavivirus)	Found in forested areas of Scandinavia. Vaccine available
Japanese B encephalitis virus — (Flavivirus)	Found in S.E. Asia. Vaccine available
Polio and enteroviruses	Most commonly cause meningitis, but meningo-encephalitis may occur
Rubella, measles viruses	Cause a subacute panencephalitis with high mortality
JC virus (Papovavirus)	Progressive multifocal leucoencephalopathy (PML) in immunocompromised
Postviral/vaccine encephalitis	Occurs with measles, influenza & others. Immune-mediated with good prognosis
Toxoplasma gondii	Occurs in immunocompromised & newborn
Cryptococcus neoformans	Commoner in AIDS patients
Plasmodium falciparum	Cerebral malaria
Trypanosoma spp.	Sleeping sickness. Occurs in central Africa
Prions	Creutzfeld–Jakob disease

TABLE 17.2

Infective causes of transverse myelitis

Cause	Disease process
Influenza and other upper respiratory tract infections Measles Rubella Mumps Vaccines	Post-infectious myelitis
Varicella-zoster virus (VZV) Human T cell lymphotropic virus (HTLV)-1 HIV *Borrelia burdoferi* (Lyme disease)	Direct infection of spinal cord
M. tuberculosis (tuberculosis) *Treponema pallidum* (syphilis) *Schistosoma* spp. (schistosomiasis)	Vasculitis of the anterior spinal artery

18 Eye infections

The exposed nature of the eye, with its warm moist environment, makes it vulnerable to a variety of microbial infections that can result in permanent loss of visual acuity or blindness (**Table 18.1**).

A cross-section of the eye with its major structures is shown in **Fig. 18.1**. Sites prone to infection are the:

- conjunctiva, producing **conjunctivitis**
- cornea, producing **keratitis**
- anterior chamber, producing intraocular **endophthalmitis**
- retina and the choroid, producing **retinochoroiditis**.

Natural defence mechanisms protect the eye from infection. The blinking action of the eyelids wipes micro-organisms from the eye surface and prevents attachment. The tearfilm that constantly bathes the external surface of the eye has antimicrobial components. These include:

- lysozyme, active against Gram-positive bacteria
- secretory IgA, which coats microbes and hampers attachment
- lactoferrin, which complexes iron and deprives bacteria of an important growth factor.

Eyelid Infection of the eyelash glands and hair follicles (**styes**) or lid margins (**blepharitis**) are common. The condition is characterised by excessive secretion of the sebaceous glands, causing a 'gritty' sensation and stickiness of the eye on waking. Bacteria are the common cause.

Conjunctiva The conjunctiva is particularly prone to infection, and **conjunctivitis** is a relatively common condition caused by bacteria, chlamydia and viruses. Symptoms are intense hyperaemia of the conjunctival vessels ('pink eye'), excessive discharge and a 'gritty' sensation in the eye. The discharge is usually watery in viral conjunctivitis or thick and purulent in bacterial conjunctivitis, resulting in 'sticky eye'.

Gonococcal neonatal conjunctivitis (**ophthalmia neonatorum**) and chlamydial **inclusion conjunctivitis** are serious conditions acquired from the female genital tract during birth. Infection can progress to keratitis, perforation and blindness. **Trachoma** is a more severe chlamydial infection that occurs in tropical countries and affects all age groups. Over 600 million people are infected world-wide, resulting in 10–20 million cases of blindness.

Cornea Viruses, bacteria, fungi, and protozoa can all cause **keratitis**. Bacteria are the most frequent cause in the northern hemisphere and fungi in the southern. Infection usually arises from direct injury to the cornea or following eye surgery. The condition can also be associated with contact lens wear. Symptoms present as a painful corneal stromal infiltrate or central abscess with overlying epithelial defect. The resulting ulcer can lead to corneal perforation and blindness. Keratitis is a serious infection, requiring prompt diagnosis, intensive antimicrobial therapy and may necessitate corneal grafting.

Intraocular **Endophthalmitis** occurs when organisms invade and multiply inside the eye chamber. The condition usually arises from accidental injury or following eye surgery (e.g. cataract removal). Bacterial flora from the eyelid and conjunctival sac are the common cause. It is therefore usual to use prophylactic topical antibiotics or antiseptics preoperatively. Rarely, endophthalmitis can arise endogenously in association with septicaemia. It is is a potentially blinding infection that can necessitate surgical removal of the eye. Prompt diagnosis and intensive intravitreal and systemic antibiotic therapy are vital in the successful treatment of the condition.

Orbital cellulitis This is an infection of the extraocular orbital tissues, resulting in painful swelling around the eye. Bacteria are the main cause, and infection usually arises from a haematogenous spread to the eye.

Retina and choroid Unlike the rest of the eye, the retina and choroid have a rich vascular supply that can result in blood-borne **retinochoroiditis**. Parasites are a common cause, as is cytomegalovirus reactivation in AIDS patients. The condition is extremely difficult to treat and may result in blindness.

Diagnosis and treatment Laboratory investigations are essential in the diagnosis and management of eye infections. This not only allows an accurate diagnosis but also, in the case of bacterial and fungal infections, provides a clinical isolate on which antibiotic sensitivity studies can be performed, enabling the appropriate choice of treatment.

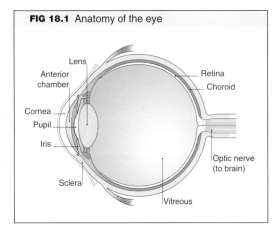

FIG 18.1 Anatomy of the eye

Lens
Anterior chamber
Cornea
Pupil
Iris
Sclera
Retina
Choroid
Optic nerve (to brain)
Vitreous

TABLE 18.1

Common microbial eye pathogens

Site	Organism	Disease	Comment	Diagnosis	Treatment
Eye margin	**Bacteria** *Staphylococcus aureus*	Styes (eye lid follicles); blepharitis (lid margin)	A common condition	Clinical appearance; swab culture	Not usually necessary; topical chloramphenicol if recurrent infection
Orbit	**Bacteria** *Haemophilus influenzae* serotype b	Cellulitis of periorbital tissues	Common in children under 5 years prior to introduction of Hib vaccine	Blood culture	Systemic antibiotics
	β-haemolytic streptococci		Affects all age groups	Ditto	Ditto
Conjunctiva	**Bacteria** *Haemophilus influenzae* *Streptococcus pneumoniae*	Conjunctivitis		Swab culture Ditto	Topical chloramphenicol Topical antibiotics (e.g. chloramphenicol)
	Neisseria gonorrhoeae	Ophthalmia neonatorum	Acquired during birth from an infected mother	Ditto	Parenteral antibiotics; topical chloramphenicol (newborn)
	Chlamydia *Chlamydia trachomatis* serotypes A–C	Trachoma; conjunctivitis and keratitis	Common in tropics; person to person transmission from contaminated flies, fingers, towels, etc.	Swab culture; immunodiagnosis	Topical tetracycline and oral erythromycin
	Chlamydia trachomatis serotypes D–K	Inclusion conjunctivitis	Acquired from birth canal of infected mother	Ditto	Ditto
	Viruses Adenovirus (serotypes 3,7,8,19)		Can spread from ophthalmic instruments and shared eye protectors ('shipyard eye')	Swab culture in mammalian cell lines	None
	Enterovirus (serotype 70) Coxsackie A (serotype 24) Measles virus			Ditto Ditto Ditto	None None None
Cornea	**Bacteria** *Pseudomonas aeruginosa*	Keratitis	Trauma, eye surgery or use of contaminated contact lens solutions	Corneal scraping culture	Topical and systemic antibiotics
	Virus Herpes simplex virus	Conjunctivitis and keratitis	Viral dormancy in ophthalmic division of the trigeminal ganglia can lead to reactivation and dendritic corneal ulcer	Corneal scraping culture in mammalian cell lines	Topical acyclovir
	Fungi *Aspergillus, Candida albicans, Fusarium* and others	Keratitis and endophthalmitis	Uncommon ocular pathogens	Corneal scraping microscopy and culture	Topical and systemic antifungal agents: e.g. ketoconazole, miconazole, amphotericin B
	Protozoa *Acanthamoeba*	Keratitis	Soil and water amoeba; most common in contact lens wearers	Corneal scraping microscopy and culture	Topical polyhexamethylene biguanide and/or propamidine isethionate
	Microsporidia	Keratitis and conjunctivitis	Recently recognised intracellular eye pathogens; mostly found in immunosuppressed persons	Corneal scraping microscopy	Albendazole
Intraocular	**Bacteria** Staphylococci and streptococci	Endophthalmitis	From flora of eyelid and conjunctival sac	Aqueous humour fluid microscopy and culture	Intravitreal and systemic antibiotics depending on organism sensitivity
	Pseudomonas aeruginosa		Can contaminate antiseptic solutions used in surgery	Ditto	
	Virus Rubella	Lens cataract (clouding) and retinochoroiditis	Acquired in utero	Serology	None
Retina and choroid	**Virus** Cytomegalovirus	Retinochoroiditis	Can be acquired in utero; reactivation in AIDS produces serious disease	Serology	Systemic/intravitreal ganciclovir or cidofovir
	Protozoa and helminths *Toxoplasma gondii*	Toxoplasmosis; retinochoroiditis	Usually acquired in utero; immunosuppression may lead to reactivation	Serology	Pyrimethamine with sulphonamides
	Toxocara canis and *cati*	Toxocariasis; retinochoroiditis	Infection from contaminated dog and cat faeces can result in ocular larval migrans (OLM)	Serology	Diethylcarbamazine, thiabendazole and mebendazole
	Onchocerca volvulus	Onchocerciasis ('river blindness'); may also involve keratitis	Transmitted by *Simulium* biting flies	Serology	Ivermectin

Viral skin rashes

19

Viruses cause rashes with four basic components (**Fig. 19.1**):

- macular/maculopapular
- vesicular/pustular
- papular/nodular
- haemorrhagic/petechial.

Enteroviruses cause rashes of any type, including vesicular rashes with a zosteriform distribution.

Macular/maculopapular rashes (Table 19.1)

Most commonly diseases of childhood, these are not true infections of the skin but **exanthems**, the primary infection occurring elsewhere with the rash as a secondary, probably immune-mediated phenomenon; virus cannot be easily, if at all, isolated from the rash. An **enanthem**, a rash on a mucous membrane, may also be detectable early in the illness; in measles these are called Koplik's spots, manifest as white flecks on the buccal mucosa. Transmission is by the respiratory route, with upper respiratory tract symptoms being common, if transient.

Measles, a paramyxovirus, can cause a severe infection with constitutional symptoms and marked upper respiratory tract symptoms. It may be complicated by secondary bacterial pneumonia, typically due to *Staphylococcus aureus*. It may also be complicated by neurological disease: acute 'post-infectious' measles encephalitis, which is immune-mediated; subacute encephalitis occurring in immunocompromised patients; rarely, subacute sclerosing panencephalitis (SSPE) occurring 5–10 years after primary infection. In children, particularly those with protein malnutrition, measles remains a common cause of death in the developing world.

Rubella may be complicated by encephalitis, haematological deficiencies and an arthritis that affects small and medium-sized joints. The most serious manifestation is, however, **congenital rubella syndrome** (neural, cardiac, bone & other abnormalities).

Confirmation of a clinical diagnosis is not usually required but can be made by culture of the virus from respiratory tract or urine (measles and rubella), or serologically (rubella, B19, HHV-6). Management of cases is symptomatic unless complicated. MMR vaccination should be instituted in early childhood.

Vesicular/pustular rashes (Table 19.2)

Chickenpox is also an infection spread by the respiratory route with an exanthem and enanthem. Initial acquisition of virus results in dormancy in the dorsal ganglia. Subsequent reduced cell-mediated immunity (as occurs in the elderly, with cancer patients or those on immunosuppressive therapy) allows the virus to track down the sensory nerve to cause a rash in the supplied dermatome: **herpes zoster**.

Recurrence of chickenpox is rare. HSV similarly exhibits latency in ganglia, with recurrence in the skin of the supplied nerve. HSV-2 has a higher recurrence rate than HSV-1.

Diagnosis of these infections is clinical, although VZV and HSV infection can be confirmed serologically. Smallpox resembled chickenpox but has now been eradicated. Aciclovir and derivatives are used in potentially complicated herpesvirus (VZV and HSV) infections, including ophthalmic infection.

The vesicles in these infections contain virus, and transmissibility is high to susceptible individuals such as the immunocompromised and newborn. Hand–foot and mouth disease is not severe, but herpesvirus infections may become disseminated, with organ damage and possible fatality. Infection control measures should be considered and exposed susceptible individuals managed with antivirals and/or, in the case of VZV infection, zoster immune-globulin.

Papular/nodular rashes (Table 19.3)

The causes of these rashes are common, infectious and, usually, non-life-threatening. The exception is specific types of HPV (mainly types 16 and 18) which are associated with cervical cancer. Diagnosis is clinical, and treatment is by physical methods such as freezing, chemicals or surgery (if warts are large). Interferon has also been used with success by injection into warts.

Haemorrhagic/petechial rashes (Table 19.4)

Some viruses uncommonly cause thrombocytopaenia which may manifest as petechiae or, less frequently, haemorrhage: EBV, Rubella virus, CMV, parvovirus B19, HIV, VZV and measles. Other clinical manifestations are usually present.

Some tropical viral haemorrhagic fever viruses (**Table 19.4**) produce widespread haemorrhage into the skin and organs by disseminated intravascular coagulation (DIC) which, in turn, results in thromboses, infarcts and increased vascular permeability. Diagnosis is by serology. Lassa fever is treatable with ribavirin.

Mucocutaneous lymph node syndrome (Kawasaki disease)

This is an acute febrile illness of children which is caused by widespread vasculitis. Its aetiology is thought to be microbial. The manifestations are conjunctivitis, desquamative erythema affecting the mouth, tongue, hands and feet, and lymphadenopathy. There is a high 'complication' rate with arthralgia, obstructive jaundice and life-threatening myocarditis. Clinical diagnosis, accompanied by electrocardiography, should be prompt so that treatment can be instituted with immunoglobulin and anti-platelet therapy.

TABLE 19.1

Macular/maculopapular viral rashes

Disease	Cause	Characteristic clinical features
Measles	Morbilli (measles) virus	Fever prior to rash, conjunctivitis, upper respiratory tract symptoms, pronounced coalescent rash
Rubella (German measles)	Rubella virus	Occipital and other lymphadenopathy; fever of short duration if present. Rash appears on face then spreads to trunk with desquamation as it fades
Erythema infectiosum	Parvovirus B19	Evanescent rash on face ('slapped cheeks'). In adults may be complicated by arthropathy. Mid-trimester infection may result in hydropic fetus/loss. May precipitate aplastic crises in haemolytic anaemia
Roseola infantum	Human herpesvirus 6	3–5 days of fever which subsides prior to rash which appears on trunk then spreads centrifugally

TABLE 19.2

Vesicular/vesicopustular viral skin rashes

Disease	Cause	Characteristic clinical features
Chickenpox	Varicella-zoster virus (VZV)	Rash appears on trunk in crops, then spreads centrifugally. Macules turn into papules which become vesicles then pustules, with several stages seen at any one time on the body. There may be intense pruritus. May be complicated by pneumonia, Reye's syndrome, encephalitis and secondary bacterial infection
Herpes zoster	Varicella-zoster virus (VZV)	Unilateral chickenpox-like rash affecting a dermatome. May result in neuralgia, particularly in elderly. Ophthalmic zoster may cause corneal scarring. Lack of cell-mediated immunity may result in disseminated zoster with generalised rash
Herpes (orolabial, genital, elsewhere), whitlow, eczema herpeticum	Herpes simplex (HSV) 1 & 2	Multiple, painful vesicles without cropping. Primary infections usually most severe with fever, regional lymphadenopathy and constitutional upset
Hand–foot and mouth	Coxsackie A, other enteroviruses	Vesicles mainly on buccal mucosa, tongue and interdigitally on the hands and feet

TABLE 19.3

Papular/nodular viral rashes

Disease	Cause	Characteristic clinical features
Warts	human papillomaviruses (over 70 types)	Usually multiple and non-pruritic
Molluscum contagiosum	Molluscum contagiosum virus	Multiple, highly infectious, pearly papules with umbilicus

TABLE 19.4

Viral haemorrhagic fevers

Disease	Virus	Animal host	Geographical distribution
Lassa fever	Lassa fever	Bush rat	W. Africa
Marburg	Marburg	Unknown	Africa
Ebola	Ebola	Unknown	C. Africa
Bolivian haemorrhagic fever	Machupo	Bush mouse	Bolivia
Haemorrhagic fever with renal syndrome (HFRS)	Hantaan	Mice, rats	S.E. Asia, Scandinavia, E. Europe
Argentinian haemorrhagic fever	Junin	Mice	Argentina
Dengue haemorrhagic fever	Dengue	Monkey/human	Africa, Asia, S. America, Caribbean
Yellow fever	Yellow fever	Monkey/human	Africa, S. America

FIG 19.1 Components of viral rashes

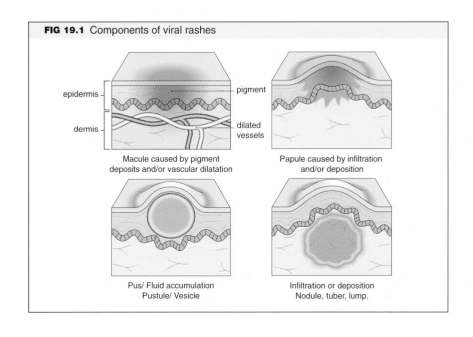

Macule caused by pigment deposits and/or vascular dilatation

Papule caused by infiltration and/or deposition

Pus/ Fluid accumulation
Pustule/ Vesicle

Infiltration or deposition
Nodule, tuber, lump.

47

20 Cutaneous infections — bacterial and fungal

The skin provides an important physical barrier to infection. In addition, the normal commensal flora helps to prevent the multiplication and invasion of pathogens. Infections of the skin and deeper tissues often follow trauma or surgery but may arise without obvious precipitating factors. As with other infections, patients with impairment of their immune system or diabetes are at greater risk.

Some infections involve only the superficial structures of the skin, whilst others affect the deeper soft tissues below the dermis (**Fig. 20.1**). The infection may be localised or spreading depending on the tissue plane involved and the virulence of the pathogen. Some of the commoner skin pathogens are shown in **Table 20.1**. In addition many systemic infections may have skin features (**Table 20.2**).

Superficial, localised infections Folliculitis is infection of the hair follicles. **Furuncles (boils)** consist of walled-off collections of organisms and associated inflammatory cells in follicles and sebaceous glands that eventually 'point' and may discharge pus. A **carbuncle** is a cluster of infected follicles commonly seen on the neck. Recurrent boils may be associated with carriage of *S. aureus* in the nose and other sites, requiring treatment with antiseptics or topical antimicrobials. **Paronychia** is infection of the tissues around the nails.

Candida infection of the skin is often associated with moist sites where skin folds rub together (**intertrigo**), e.g. the nappy area in children. **Ringworm** (tinea) is a localised infection of the epithelium caused by dermatophyte fungi. These arise from human, animal or soil sources and infect skin and hair to produce circular scaly lesions (**Fig. 20.2**).

Wound infections and abscesses Traumatic and surgical wounds may develop localised or spreading infections. Necrotic tissue or foreign materials (including sutures) act as a focus for infection. Localised walled-off infection leads to the formation of an abscess.

Animal bites Bites and scratches from dogs, cats, other pets and wild animals may lead to local or systemic bacterial infections, including cat-scratch disease caused by *Bartonella henselae*.

Spreading infections Impetigo is infection limited to the epidermis, presenting as yellow crusting lesions, most often on the face in young children. When the dermis is infected, a red demarcated rash appears called **erysipelas**. Infection spreading beneath the dermis to involve the subcutaneous fat is **cellulitis**. This severe condition may occur at any site but commonly involves the legs and presents with a demarcated red lesion often with blisters. The patient is usually systemically unwell and febrile. '**Scalded skin syndrome**' is an acute infection of babies and young children. Staphylococcal toxin causes splitting within the epidermis, leading to large areas of skin loss.

Death of tissue leads to gangrene. **Synergistic gangrene** generally affects the groin and genitals and is confined to the skin. Widespread necrosis of deeper tissues is seen in **necrotizing fasciitis** caused by 'flesh-eating bugs'. Both conditions require extensive debridement to avoid a fatal outcome. Some organisms release gas into the tissue (**gas gangrene**) which may be detected clinically as crepitus or seen in soft tissue X-rays. This typically follows trauma, ischaemia or contaminated surgery such as lower-limb amputation.

Mycobacterial infections of the skin Primary infection of the skin with *M. tuberculosis* (lupus vulgaris) is rare, but subcutaneous infection, particularly of cervical lymph nodes, is well recognised. Atypical mycobacteria cause skin infections, notably *M. marinum* which is associated with '**fish-tank**' or '**swimming pool**' **granuloma**. Tuberculoid **leprosy** causes red anaesthetic lesions on the face, body and limbs. Lepromatous leprosy is associated with destruction of the nose and maxilla.

Investigations and treatment Whilst pus or swabs may be adequate for superficial infections, tissue should be sent wherever possible. In systemic disease, blood cultures are essential. Adequate treatment requires drainage of pus and debridement of devitalised tissue in addition to appropriate antimicrobials (**Table 20.1**).

Animal bites, human bites and 'clenched fist injuries' must be carefully explored, and prophylaxis started, without delay.

Dermatophyte culture may take several weeks, and the diagnosis is often confirmed initially by the demonstration of fungal hyphae in skin scrapes or nail clippings. Many superficial fungal infections respond to topical agents, but infections of hair and nails require oral antifungals.

TABLE 20.1

Common bacterial and fungal pathogens

Pathogen	Infection	Treatment
Staph. aureus	Folliculitis, furuncles, carbuncles Wound infection/abscess Impetigo Cellulitis Scalded skin syndrome	Flucloxacillin
Strep. pyogenes	Erysipelas Impetigo Cellulitis Necrotising fasciitis	Penicillin
Mixed organisms: anaerobes, streptococci, *Staph. aureus*, Gram-negative rods	Cellulitis Necrotising fasciitis Synergistic gangrene	Cefuroxime & metronidazole +/– gentamicin
Clostridium spp.	Gas gangrene	Penicillin and/or metronidazole
Pasteurella multocida (+/– staphylococci, streptococci, anaerobes)	Cat and dog bites	Co-amoxiclav
Candida albicans	Intertrigo, paronychia	Topical clotrimazole
Dermatophytes	Ringworm (tinea)	Topical clotrimazole, oral griseofulvin or terbinafine
Malassezia furfur	Pityriasis versicolor	Topical selenium sulphide or terbinafine or oral itraconazole

TABLE 20.2

Systemic bacterial infections with skin features

Infection	Organism	Skin feature
Meningococcal septicaemia	*Neisseria meningitidis*	Petechial rash
Toxic shock syndrome	*Staph. aureus*	Rash and desquamation
Scarlet fever	*Strep. pyogenes*	Erythematous rash
Enteric fever	*Salmonella typhi* *Salmonella paratyphi*	'Rose spots'
Infective endocarditis	Streptococci *Staph. aureus*	Petechiae, splinter haemorrhages
Lyme disease	*Borrelia burgdorferi*	Erythema chronicum migrans
Septicaemia	*Pseudomonas aeruginosa*	Ecthyma gangrenosum
Syphilis	*Treponema pallidum*	Disseminated rash in second stage

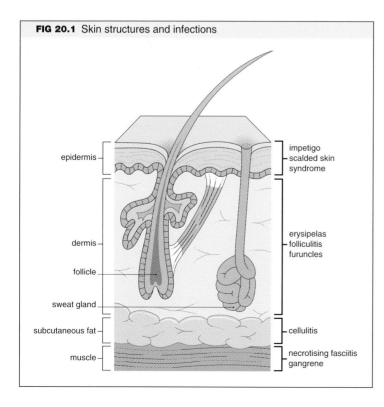

FIG 20.1 Skin structures and infections

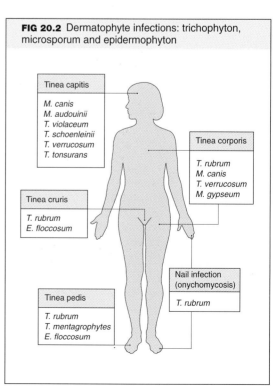

FIG 20.2 Dermatophyte infections: trichophyton, microsporum and epidermophyton

21 Gastrointestinal infections

Gastrointestinal tract infections are among the most commonly reported disease throughout the world, causing considerable morbidity and mortality. Although most prevalent in countries where sanitation and drinking water quality are poor, intestinal infections are common in the United Kingdom, and surveys indicate that the incidence is rising.

All parts of the gastrointestinal tract are susceptible to infection by a variety of micro-organisms (**Table 21.1**), and, with the exception of certain nematodes that penetrate the skin, infection arises from ingestion:

- directly from an infected human or animal by hand to mouth (faecal-oral)
- indirectly from contaminated food or water
- by consumption of food in which microbes have multiplied (food-poisoning).

Although the gastrointestinal tract is vulnerable to infection, it is also well defended. The acidity of the stomach fluids (pH 2.0) is a barrier to most microbes and stops entry of pathogens into the intestinal tract. The small and large intestine are rich in commensal bacterial flora that prevent pathogen colonisation (the colon may contain 10^{12} bacteria/g of faeces). Secretory IgA and lymphoid tissue (Peyer's patches) in the small intestine also provide immune protection.

Gastroenteritis Infection of the gastrointestinal tract results in **gastroenteritis** and refers to a collection of symptoms that include nausea, vomiting, diarrhoea and abdominal discomfort. Symptoms vary with the type of organism and health of the person. The young, old or immunosuppressed are particularly susceptible to severe illness, which may be life-threatening.

Infections are usually confined to the intestinal mucosa, but some organisms invade through the gut wall and disseminate into the blood stream, causing fever (e.g. typhoid). Diarrhoea is a natural response by the body to expel the pathogen and is usually due to infection within the small intestine. It does, however, also aid the spread of the organism and infection of others. **Dysentery** is an inflammatory disorder of the gastrointestinal tract associated with blood and pus in the faeces, fever and pain, usually resulting from infection of the large intestine. **Enterocolitis** is inflammation of both the small and large intestine.

Bacterial infections are generally slow in onset, producing diarrhoea without vomiting that may last for a week or more. In contrast, viral infections have a short incubation period and often produce both diarrhoea and vomiting which resolves within a day or two.

Food-poisoning Food is a common means by which pathogens can infect the gastrointestinal tract, usually as a result of contamination by an infected person during preparation. Alternatively, the organisms may be part of an animal's normal flora and contaminate the food during slaughtering and processing. However, in true food-poisoning, bacteria actively multiply in the food. This does not necessarily result in spoiling of the food, which appears fit for consumption and hence increases the challenge dose and likelihood of infection.

Symptoms typically include both diarrhoea and vomiting and result either directly from the presence of live bacteria or from toxins produced in the food during growth (**Table 21.2**). The time between food consumption and onset of symptoms can indicate the likely cause in food-poisoning (**Table 21.1**).

Antibiotic-associated diarrhoea Certain antibiotics with broad-spectrum activity can seriously disturb the normal flora of the gut. *Clostridium difficile*, part of the gut flora in low numbers, can flourish under such circumstances. This may result in a severe infection termed **pseudomembranous colitis** due to toxin production by the bacterium. Hospitalised elderly patients are particularly prone to infection.

Peptic ulceration The bacterium *Helicobacter pylori* has recently been implicated as a cause of chronic gastritis and peptic ulcer disease. The pathogenesis of helicobacter-associated peptic ulcers is still being investigated, although a direct link between the bacterium and gastric disease is now accepted.

Diagnosis and treatment Intestinal infections are diagnosed by the detection of organisms in faecal specimens: electron microscopy, immunoassay or gene detection for viruses; culture and biochemical identification of bacteria; microscopy and immunoassays for protozoa and helminths.

Antibiotic treatment is not usually indicated in viral and bacterial gastrointestinal infections except in severe cases, as this only prolongs symptoms and encourages drug resistance. Exceptions are in pseudomembranous colitis, helicobacter-associated peptic ulcers and typhoid fever. Antiprotozoal and antihelminthic agents are usually necessary in parasite infections.

TABLE 21.1

Common causes of gastroenteritis

Pathogen	Incubation time	Duration	Diarrhoea	Vomiting	Pain	Fever
Bacteria						
Bacillus cereus toxin	1–6 h	2–24 h	+	+++	–	–
Campylobacter	2–11 days	3 days–3 weeks	+++	–	++	++
Clostridium botulinum toxin (botulism)	22–>48 h	weeks–months	–	(+)	–	–
Clostridium difficile (pseudomembranous colitis)	3–4 days	several weeks	++	–	+	+/–
Clostridium perfringens toxin	18–36 h	24 h – 3 days	+	++	+	–
Verotoxigenic *E. coli* (VTEC)	1–5 days	3–5 days	++	+	++	+
Enterotoxigenic *E. coli* (ETEC)	1–5 days	3–5 days	+++	(+)	++	+
Helicobacter pylori (gastritis and peptic ulcers)	Unknown	Several weeks (with treatment) or chronic carriage	–	–	+	–
Salmonella (salmonellosis)	18–36 h	48 h – 7 days	++	+	–	+
Salmonella typhi and *paratyphi* (typhoid and paratyphoid fever)	7–21 days	4–6 weeks or chronic carriage	(+)	–	–	++
Shigella (bacillary dysentery)	1–4 days	2–3 days	+++	–	+	+
Staphylococcus aureus toxin	0.5–6 h	2–12 h	(+)	+++	–	–
Vibrio cholerae (cholera)	2–3 days	1–7 days	++++	+	–	–
Vibrio parahaemolyticus	8 h – 2 days	3 days	++	+	+	+
Yersinia enterocolitica	4–7 days	1–2 weeks	++	–	++	+
Viruses						
Adenovirus (types 40,41)	2–4 days	1–2 days	++	+	+	–
Astrovirus	1–2 days	1–2 days	++	+	–	–
Calicivirus	16–24 h	1–2 days	+	++	–	+
Norwalk virus	1–3 days	1–2 days	+	++	–	–
Rotavirus	1–3 days	2–5 days	++	++	–	–
Protozoa						
Cryptosporidium parvum (cryptosporidiosis)	3–6 days	immunocompetent: 7–21 days	++	–	–	(+)
		immunocompromised: chronic	+++	–	–	(+)
Entamoeba histolytica (amoebiasis)	days–weeks	7–14 days or chronic carriage	++	–	++	+
Giardia lamblia (giardiasis)	5–21 days	7–10 days or chronic carriage	+	–	+	–

Helminths

Ascaris lumbricoides, Enterobius vermicularis, Trichuris trichuria, hookworms, *Strongyloides stercoralis, Trichinella spiralis, Toxocara*	These helminths infect the gut as part of their life cycles. However, they do not usually cause symptoms of gastroenteritis. Further details are given elsewhere (see Chapter 6)

TABLE 21.2

Common causes of food-poisoning

Pathogen	Common food source	Comment
Organisms capable of replicating in food		
Salmonella	Poultry, eggs	Present in the gut of poultry and cattle
Bacillus cereus toxin	Reheated rice	Spores germinate on reheating, releasing heat-resistant toxins
Clostridium perfringens toxin	Reheated meat foods (gravy, stews, pies, large joints, etc.)	Spores germinate on reheating, and replicating bacteria are ingested, releasing toxins in the gut
Clostridium botulinum toxin (botulism)	Inadequately canned foods, home preserved fruits and vegetables	Spores germinate under anaerobic storage conditions, releasing a paralysing neuromuscular toxin
Staphylococcus aureus toxin	Meat and dairy products	Results by food contamination from an infected individual (boils, wounds, nasal and skin carriage)
Organisms commonly transmitted in food		
Campylobacter	Poultry, unpasteurised milk	Commonest cause of bacterial gastroenteritis in UK (40 000 cases a year and rising)
Verotoxigenic *E. coli* (VTEC)[a]	Meat (notably hamburgers), unpasteurised milk, any food contaminated with faeces	Present in beef and dairy cattle and of increasing importance in UK (notably serotype O157)
Yersinia enterocolitica	Raw or undercooked pork	Rare in UK but common in other European countries
Vibrio parahaemolyticus	Filter-feeding shellfish	Bacterium is concentrated within shell-fish; rare in UK
Aeromonas	Freshwater fish	Common in aquatic environments and has been isolated from faeces of some symptomatic persons

[a]VTEC toxin acts on gut mucosa, causing a bloody diarrhoea (**haemorrhagic colitis**) or systemically, resulting in haemolysis and renal failure (**haemolytic uraemic syndrome**)

22 Hepatitis and pancreatitis

Infection of the liver and pancreas occurs via the blood stream, rarely from the gastrointestinal tract, even when the route of acquisition is faecal-oral. Biliary tract infection and peritonitis are, conversely, due to locally spread infection.

Hepatitis The classic clinical triad of jaundice, dark urine and pale stools accompanying fever is often missing, particularly in children, who are more often asymptomatic. The vast majority of cases are of viral aetiology, with hepatitis A, B and C being the commonest (**Table 22.1**). Diagnosis of viral (and leptospiral) infection is serological, by either detection of antigen or specific antibody.

The detection of hepatitis B surface antigen (HBsAg) confirms the diagnosis of hepatitis B virus, and the presence of hepatitis B 'e' antigen (HBeAg) indicates a high infectious risk. Other markers are determined in specific cases (**Fig. 22.1**). Jaundice in carriers, in whom HBsAg persists for 6 months or more, is most likely to have another cause, which should be sought. Hepatitis A virus (HAV) infection is diagnosed by anti-HAV IgM. Serological assays for the diagnosis of hepatitis C do not offer early diagnosis, as they are based on the detection of specific IgG, which may take several weeks; diagnosis is thus retrospective but can be made early by gene amplification methods such as PCR.

Management of acute viral hepatitis is supportive, with bed rest at the peak of liver inflammation. Chronic hepatitis therapy is evolving, with drugs such as interferon, immunomodulators and ribavirin being used with moderate success in delaying progression of liver disease, although viral eradication is not achieved. Prevention of infection involves public health measures and vaccination for hepatitis A and hepatitis B. Travellers from the UK to higher-prevalence areas (outside northern and western Europe and North America) should consider vaccination for hepatitis A. Although universal vaccination for hepatitis B is being introduced in several countries, in the UK it is targeted at higher-risk groups, such as medical, nursing and laboratory staff, 'gay' men, and residents of mental institutions. In the event of contacts with both hepatitis A and hepatitis B, passive immunisation is available for susceptible individuals.

About 10% of cases of hepatitis do not have an identifiable cause, and new viruses such as hepatitis G and TT virus have been discovered by modern molecular methods in some cases. Their aetiological role has, however, yet to be defined.

Liver abscess These may be primary infections or secondary to haematogenous spread from another site. Usually bacterial, with mixed anaerobic and aerobic flora (including Enterobacteriaceae and *Streptococcus milleri* group), they consist of pus that has been walled off by a fibrinous layer; this can be detected by imaging. Single lesions are often asymptomatic unless very large. Broad-spectrum antibiotics are used to treat the condition, but surgical drainage may also be required.

Biliary tract infection This occurs secondary to obstruction — either gallstones or malignancy. Ascending cholangitis, liver abscess and septicaemia may be sequelae. Diagnosis is clinical, with imaging used as a confirmatory test. Treatment consists of removal of the obstruction and broad-spectrum antibiotics.

Peritonitis Contamination of the sterile peritoneal cavity occurs through breach of the bowel or urogenital wall. This may be iatrogenic, such as occurs in surgery, or through diseases such as inflammatory bowel disease, appendicitis and malignancy. Occasionally tuberculosis or actinomycosis of the genital tract may have been the initial site of infection. Genital chlamydia and gonococcal infections can also ascend to cause perihepatitis (so-called **FitzHugh–Curtis syndrome**). Clinical diagnosis is confirmed operatively, or through laparoscopy, with pus and/or adhesions visible between the peritoneal layers. Treatment with broad-spectrum antibiotics may be required, as infections arising from the gut are polymicrobial.

Pancreatitis This can be caused by a number of viruses (**Table 22.2**). Mumps is the commonest. Diabetes mellitus is associated with preceding enterovirus infection. Bacteria can cause pancreatitis, with mixed flora, if there is obstruction at the ampulla of Vater, usually due to malignancy.

TABLE 22.1

Infective causes of hepatitis

Cause	Route of transmission	Characteristic features
Hepatitis A	Faecal-oral	Incubation period of 2–4 weeks. <1% of cases are fulminant
Hepatitis B	Blood-borne	Incubation period of 1–3 months. Immune complex form and may cause arthralgia, urticarial rash and glomerulonephritis. 10% become chronic carriers, with subsequent chronic hepatitis, cirrhosis and hepatocellular carcinoma. High prevalence of infection, carriage and hepatoma in S.E. Asia
Hepatitis C	Blood-borne	Incubation period of 2–4 months. 90% become carriers
Hepatitis D	Blood-borne	Defective virus requiring hepatitis B or herpes simplex to replicate. Co-infection with hepatitis B makes it more severe; super-infection results in recurrence
Hepatitis E	Faecal-oral	Incubation period 6–8 weeks. Water-borne epidemics have been seen in India and the former Soviet Union, with 20% mortality in pregnant women in 3rd trimester due to disseminated intravascular coagulation
Leptospira interrogans (leptospirosis, Weils' disease)	Faecal-oral	Spirochaetes can also enter through skin. Sewerage workers at risk from infected rat urine. May be complicated by aseptic meningitis and haemorrhages. Treatment is with penicillin
Entamoeba histolytica (amoebiasis)		Causes pseudoabscess
Parasitic infections (schistosomiasis, clonorchiasis, fascioliasis)	Faecal-oral	Infections of mainly tropical climates
Others (CMV, EBV, HSV, rubella, yellow fever, TB, toxoplasmosis, syphilis, etc.)	Various	Usually part of generalised infection

TABLE 22.2

Infective causes of acute pancreatitis

Mumps
Enteroviruses
Cytomegalovirus
Epstein–Barr virus
Mixed bacterial flora

FIG 22.1 Time course of markers in hepatitis B infection

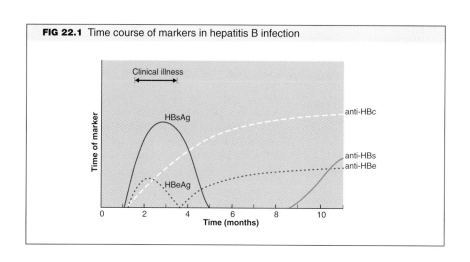

23 Infections of the heart

Endocarditis is an uncommon but serious disease involving the endothelial lining of the heart, particularly the cardiac valves. Even with appropriate therapy there is a mortality rate of up to 30% — untreated mortality approaches 100%. In many patients, predisposing factors are found such as:

- congenital heart disease
- rheumatic heart disease
- degenerative heart disease
- other cardiac lesions, e.g. mitral valve prolapse
- i.v. drug usage
- prosthetic heart valve.

Native valve endocarditis is distinguished from **prosthetic valve endocarditis**, which can be divided into early (occurring within 2 months of surgery) or late onset.

The majority of cases of endocarditis are caused by bacteria, although fungi and other organisms are sometimes implicated (**Table 23.1**). Organisms reach the valves following **bacteraemia** which may arise from a number of sources including dental procedures (e.g. extractions, scaling or even vigorous brushing), invasive instrumentation (e.g. bronchoscopy) or surgery of the gastrointestinal or genitourinary tracts. **Adherence** of organisms is enhanced by the presence of fibrin-platelet deposits on damaged endothelium and by bacterial factors such as adhesins and fibronectin-binding proteins. The accumulation of fibrin, platelets and organisms forms **vegetations** that may interfere with valvular function or form **emboli** to distant organs.

The onset of endocarditis may be insidious and the diagnosis difficult, but the following **clinical features** may suggest the diagnosis:

- fever (often low-grade)
- general malaise with anorexia and weight loss
- new or changing heart murmurs
- embolic phenomena (especially skin and brain)
- immune complex disease (nephritis and some skin lesions, e.g. splinter haemorrhages).

Investigations The haemoglobin may be reduced and white cell count and markers of an acute phase response such as plasma viscosity and C-reactive protein increased. Haematuria and proteinuria should be sought to indicate nephritis. Vegetations may be detected at transthoracic **echocardiography**, although transoesophageal examinations are more sensitive, particularly in prosthetic valve disease (**Fig. 23.1**).

An essential element of diagnosis is **blood culture**, which should be undertaken before starting antimicrobial therapy. Three cultures should be taken from separate venepunctures at different times within 24 h. Scrupulous aseptic technique is essential, as skin organisms are generally contaminants but are also common

pathogens in prosthetic valve endocarditis. **Culture-negative endocarditis** may be due to prior antimicrobial treatment or fastidious organisms that require special culture techniques or serology for their detection. Surgical material (valves, vegetations, pus, etc.) should be examined carefully by microscopy and culture.

Management The importance of obtaining an isolate is that detailed susceptibility studies are important in optimising antimicrobial treatment. The **minimum inhibitory concentration (MIC)** of antibacterials should be determined to ensure appropriate doses and duration of therapy. In most cases combination therapy is employed to provide enhanced activity: e.g. the addition of gentamicin to benzylpenicillin improves bactericidal activity against many streptococci and enterococci.

High-dose regimens for several weeks are required for successful therapy, and clinicians should liaise closely with microbiologists to select and monitor therapy. Antibiotic levels (e.g. gentamicin, vancomycin) need monitoring closely, and serial measurements of C-reactive protein (together with temperature, white cell count and plasma viscosity) are helpful in assessing response.

Where extensive valvular damage has occurred (and in most cases of prosthetic disease), valve replacement may be required in addition to antimicrobial therapy.

Prophylaxis As bacteraemia may result in endocarditis in susceptible patients, prophylactic regimens are recommended for

- dental procedures
- genitourinary surgery or instrumentation
- gastrointestinal procedures
- obstetric and gynaecological procedures.

These regimens are based on consensus statements and experimental evidence, as the incidence of endocarditis is too low to conduct controlled trials. Current detailed advice is given in the *British National Formulary*.

Myocarditis and pericarditis Infection of the heart muscle or pericardium is often viral in origin, although pericarditis may present as a severe bacterial infection (**Table 23.2**). Typical symptoms include a 'flu'-like illness and localised pain. Myocarditis may cause dysrhythmia and, in severe cases, heart failure. In pericarditis a pericardial rub may be heard, and in severe cases, typically caused by pyogenic bacteria, effusion may be demonstrated by chest X-ray or echocardiography. Respiratory swabs and stool samples should be cultured for viruses, and blood and pericardial fluid (where available) cultured for bacteria. Viral infections are usually self-limiting, but bacterial infections require prompt treatment.

TABLE 23.1

Causative organisms in endocarditis

Organisms	Comments	Typical treatment
Viridans streptococci	Oral commensal flora: examples include *Strep. sanguis*, *Strep. mitior*, *Strep. mutans*, *Strep. milleri* group. Commonest cause in native valve disease and late prosthetic valve endocarditis	Benzylpenicillin +/− gentamicin
Enterococci	Usually *E. faecalis*. Often bowel/urinary tract source	Ampicillin + gentamicin
Staphylococcus aureus	Acute and destructive endocarditis. More common in i.v. drug users	Flucloxacillin +/− gentamicin
Coagulase-negative staphylococci	Commonest cause of early prosthetic valve disease. Rare in natural valve disease	Vancomycin + rifampicin
Gram-negative bacilli	Includes some oral commensal bacteria. Enteric bacteria rare in natural valve disease, but occasionally seen in i.v. drug users and prosthetic disease	As dictated by sensitivities
Fungi	Mainly *Candida* species. Generally associated with i.v. drug users and prosthetic valve disease	Fluconazole or amphotericin
Coxiella burnetii	Q fever. Usually diagnosed serologically	Tetracycline

FIG 23.1 Aortic vegetation seen on echocardiography

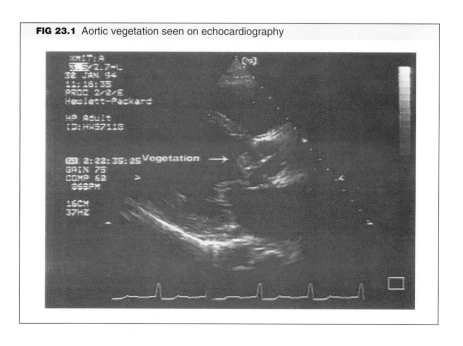

TABLE 23.2

Pathogens in myocarditis and pericarditis

Myocarditis	Pericarditis
Viruses	
Enteroviruses, especially coxsackie	Enteroviruses, especially coxsackie
Echovirus	Influenza A & B
Influenza A & B	
Rubella	
Epstein–Barr virus	
Cytomegalovirus	
Bacteria	
Coxiella burnetii	*Mycoplasma pneumoniae*
Leptospira spp.	*Strep. pneumoniae*
Mycoplasma pneumoniae	*Strep. pyogenes*
N. meningitidis	*Staph. aureus*
	Mycobacterium tuberculosis
	Coxiella burnetii

24 Urinary tract infections

Urinary tract infections are more common at certain ages in males and females (**Fig. 24.1**). Whilst many infections are mild, renal infections may lead to long-term renal damage, and the urinary tract is a common source of life-threatening Gram-negative bacteraemia. Several clinical syndromes are recognised (**Table 24.1**), the commonest being lower urinary tract infection of the bladder (**cystitis**). Upper urinary tract infection (**pyelonephritis**) may result from haematogenous or ascending routes of infection.

Pathogenesis

The pathogenesis of urinary tract infections is summarised in (**Table 24.2**). The additional risk factors (including instrumentation and catheterisation) in hospitalised patients lead to a difference in the organisms isolated (**Fig. 24.2**).

The normal urinary tract is sterile, but urine may be contaminated with organisms from the distal urethra during voiding. Kass defined the term **significant bacteriuria** as $>10^5$ colony-forming units (cfu) of a single organism per millilitre of urine. This figure was derived from studies in women and was found to distinguish pyelonephritis from contamination. However, despite regular usage since, this figure is not validated for other urinary infections or those in men or children. In patients with symptomatic infections, counts may be as low as 10^2 cfu/ml.

About 50% of women who present with the clinical features of cystitis do not have positive urine cultures, a condition known as abacterial cystitis or 'urethral syndrome'. The aetiology of this condition is controversial, but explanations include:

- infection with low counts of bacteria
- infection with fastidious organisms not detected on routine culture
- sexually transmitted infections, e.g. chlamydia
- non-infective inflammation, e.g. chemical.

Asymptomatic bacteriuria occurs in about 5% of women and is important in pregnancy, where, untreated, 20–30% of cases will develop acute pyelonephritis. Bacteriuria in pregnancy is also associated with premature birth, low birth weight and increased perinatal mortality. It is therefore important that all women have their urine cultured early in pregnancy.

Microbiological investigations and interpretation

Urine specimens need to be collected with care to minimise contamination with periurethral organisms. The first portion of voided urine is discarded and a **midstream urine (MSU)** specimen collected. Specimens from catheterised patients should be collected by needle aspiration from the catheter tubing. In children specimens may be collected in adhesive bags, but, to avoid contamination, suprapubic aspiration may be required. Where there may be a delay in examination, specimens should be refrigerated or collected in containers with boric acid to prevent bacterial multiplication in transit. Microscopy for white and red blood cells may be helpful in the interpretation of culture results, but their presence does not necessarily indicate urinary tract infection. Squamous epithelial cells usually indicate contamination of the specimen. Quantitative culture is followed by susceptibility testing of significant isolates. Some clinicians and laboratories use **screening methods** to exclude urinary infection. Dipstick tests are available for the detection of blood, leucocyte esterase (indicating white blood cells) and nitrite (indicating the presence of nitrate-reducing bacteria).

The interpretation of culture results depends on clinical details (symptoms, previous antibiotics), quality of specimen, delay in culture and species isolated. Repeat specimens may be required with low bacterial counts, evidence of contamination or so-called 'sterile pyuria' — white blood cells in the urine without bacterial growth. This may be caused by:

- prior antibiotics
- urethritis (chlamydia or gonococci)
- vaginal infection or inflammation
- fastidious organisms (controversial significance)
- non-infective inflammation (e.g. tumours, chemicals)
- urinary tuberculosis.

Where **tuberculosis** is considered, three early morning urine specimens should be collected for culture when the urine is most concentrated.

Treatment

Uncomplicated cystitis should be treated with a short (typically 3 day) course of an oral antibacterial agent such as trimethoprim or nitrofurantoin. Post-treatment **follow-up cultures** are particularly important in children and pregnant women. For patients with complicated infections, antibiotics such as cephalosporins or gentamicin are often indicated depending on antibiotic susceptibility (**Fig. 24.3**). In catheterised patients, antimicrobial treatment is usually only recommended in patients with systemic features. The catheter should be removed whenever possible. Pyelonephritis requires treatment, initially systemic, for a total of 10–14 days.

In selected cases a prophylactic dose of an antibacterial agent given at night may reduce the incidence of recurrent cystitis.

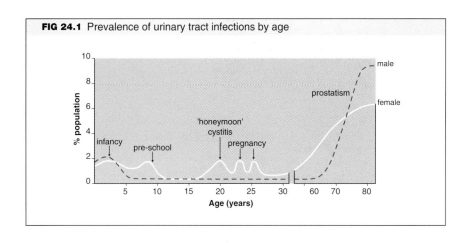

FIG 24.1 Prevalence of urinary tract infections by age

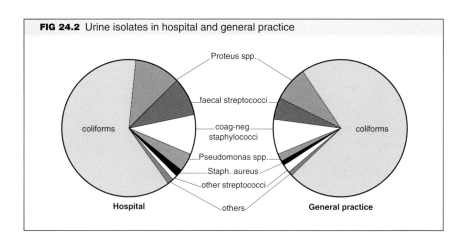

FIG 24.2 Urine isolates in hospital and general practice

Proteus spp.

faecal streptococci

coag-neg
staphylococci

Pseudomonas spp.

Staph. aureus

other streptococci

coliforms

coliforms

others

Hospital

General practice

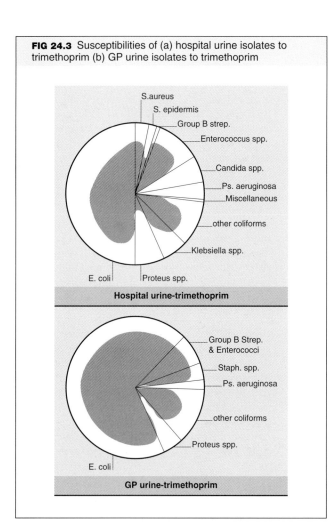

FIG 24.3 Susceptibilities of (a) hospital urine isolates to trimethoprim (b) GP urine isolates to trimethoprim

S.aureus
S. epidermis
Group B strep.
Enterococcus spp.
Candida spp.
Ps. aeruginosa
Miscellaneous
other coliforms
Klebsiella spp.
E. coli
Proteus spp.

Hospital urine-trimethoprim

Group B Strep.
& Enterococci
Staph. spp.
Ps. aeruginosa
other coliforms
Proteus spp.
E. coli

GP urine-trimethoprim

TABLE 24.1

Clinical syndromes of the urinary tract

Lower urinary tract

Bacterial cystitis	Frequency and dysuria, often with pyuria and haematuria
Abacterial cystitis	As above but without 'significant bacteriuria'
Prostatitis	Fever, dysuria, frequency with perineal and low back pain

Upper urinary tract

Acute pyelonephritis	Symptoms of cystitis plus fever and loin pain
Chronic interstitial nephritis	Renal impairment following chronic inflammation — infection one of many causes

Asymptomatic

Covert bacteriuria	Detected only by culture. Important in children and pregnancy

TABLE 24.2

Pathogenesis of urinary tract infections

Host factors

Shorter urethra	More infections in females
Obstruction	Enlarged prostate, pregnancy, stones, tumours
Neurological problems	Incomplete emptying, residual urine
Ureteric reflux	Ascending infection from bladder, especially in children

Bacterial factors

Faecal flora	Potential urinary pathogens colonise periurethral area
Adhesion	Fimbriae and adhesins allow attachment to urethral and bladder epithelium
K antigens	Allow some *E. coli* to resist host defences by producing polysaccharide capsule
Haemolysins	Damage membranes and cause renal damage
Urease	Produced by some bacteria, e.g. *Proteus*

25 Genital tract infections

This category includes a number of sexually transmitted diseases (STDs) that affect the genital tract, as well as some infections that do not require sexual activity for transmission (**Fig. 25.1**). Sexually transmissible infections whose main symptoms occur outside the genital tract, e.g. HIV and Hepatitis B, are considered elsewhere. STDs require intimate contact for transmission, the rates generally being highest from male to female. The site of infection will depend upon the nature of the sexual act that was performed. Contact tracing is undertaken following diagnosis of an STD to reduce transmission within the community, and, for this reason, general practitioners will often refer patients to the local genitourinary clinic where all the facilities are available. Having declined in recent years, probably because of individuals' precautions against HIV infection, the rates of all STDs now appear to be rising again. The laboratory methods of diagnosis and the treatments for genital infections are summarised in **Table 25.1**.

In the male, with the exception of the distal 2–3 cm, the normal urethra is sterile, protected by mucus, prostatic secretions and periodic flushing with urine. The commensal flora of the vagina offers some protective effect in the female, as does the mucus within the cervix and the uterine cell turnover through menstruation.

Skin infections (both sexes)

Herpes simplex is a relapsing condition that produces multiple painful ulcers on the genital skin and mucous membranes following a variable prodrome of tingling. Human papilloma virus infection is generally a self-limiting condition marked by non-painful warts or dry scaling lesions on the genital skin; although it is less obvious, mucosal surfaces may also be infected with certain types of virus, bringing an increased risk of carcinoma, particularly of the cervix.

Syphilis is a multisystem disorder diagnosed serologically and caused by the bacterial spirochaete *Treponema pallidum*. The disease is now rare.

More common in the tropics are three ulcerative conditions with regional lymphadenopathy — chancroid, granuloma inguinale, lymphogranuloma venereum — caused by *H. ducreyi, Calymmatobacterium granulomatis,* and *Chlamydia trachomatis* serotypes L1–L3, respectively.

Infection in the male

Urethritis in males is usually symptomatic, with discharge and dysuria. *C. trachomatis* serotypes D–K are the most common cause, although more severe symptoms suggests infection with *N. gonorrhoeae*. Mixed infections are common. Urethritis may progress to involve the prostate or epididymis, which may be more difficult to treat. Reiter's syndrome (urethritis, iritis and arthritis) is an unpleasant relapsing condition that may follow an episode of urethritis, particularly in HLA B27 carriers.

Proctitis is most common amongst male homosexuals, with rectal pain, bleeding and discharge. Apart from the known causes listed in **Fig. 25.1**, other changes in bowel flora occur (e.g. the acquisition of novel *Campylobacter* species) the significance of which is unclear.

Infection in the female

Silent infections are common in women.

N. gonorrhoeae may cause infection of Bartholin's glands at the vaginal introitus, although other bacteria can also be responsible. Vaginal discharge is a common reason for medical consultation, and an accurate diagnosis may usually be obtained in the surgery from a vaginal swab using the features described in **Table 25.2**. Candidiasis is a very common problem that is more likely with the contraceptive pill, pregnancy, diabetes and following the use of antibiotics. Similarly, **anaerobic** or **bacterial vaginosis** is caused by a disturbance in the normal vaginal flora, often following the use of broad-spectrum antibiotics.

If the problem is seen to arise from the cervical os and not the vagina, samples of the discharge should be sent to the microbiology laboratory for more-detailed analysis. The causes of cervical infection are all sexually transmitted, with chlamydia being the most common. Whilst infection may often be asymptomatic, it is still a reservoir for spread to others through sexual contact and for ascending infection.

Pelvic inflammatory disease (PID) may present as an acute peritonitis, as chronic pelvic pain and dyspareunia or be clinically silent. Regardless of the presentation, there is a significant risk of damage to the Fallopian tubes, leading to an increased incidence of ectopic pregnancy and infertility. Treatment will often involve the 'blind' use of antibiotics, as a microbiological diagnosis is unlikely unless laparoscopy is performed.

TABLE 25.1

Detection and treatment of genital tract infection

Infectious agent	Method of detection	Treatment of choice
Herpes simplex virus[a]	Clinical, viral culture, electron microscopy	Aciclovir or related drug
Human papilloma virus[a]	Clinical only	Chemical or surgical removal
N. gonorrhoeae[a]	Culture, microscopy, DNA amplification	Ciprofloxacin, 3rd generation cephalosporin, azithromycin
C. trachomatis[a]	Antigen detection, DNA amplification, (tissue culture)	Tetracycline, azithromycin
Mycoplasma genitalium	Culture	Tetracycline
T. pallidum[a]	Antibody detection	Penicillin
Anaerobic vaginosis	Culture, microscopy	Metronidazole, (co-amoxyclav)
(Gardnerella vaginalis anaerobes)		
Haemophilus ducreyi	Microscopy & culture	Erythromycin
Calymmatobacterium granulomatis	Culture	Tetracycline
Candida spp.	Microscopy, culture	Fluconazole, (nystatin)
Trichomonas vaginalis[a]	Microscopy, culture	Metronidazole

[a]Sexually transmitted diseases

TABLE 25.2

Discharge from the female genital tract

Infection/condition	Site	pH	KOH	Microscopy	Clinical features
Normal	Vagina	< 4.5	–	Lactobacilli	Minimal discharge, variable colour
Candidiasis	Vagina	< 4.5	–	Budding yeasts/hyphae	Yellowish-white discharge/plaques, pruritus
Trichomoniasis	Vagina	> 4.5	Malodour ++	Motile parasites	Profuse frothy foul-smelling yellow-green discharge, vaginal petechiae
Bacterial vaginosis	Vagina	> 4.5	Malodour +++	Clue cells Gram-negative bacilli	Foul-smelling grey-white discharge, pruritus, dyspareunia
Gonorrhoea	Cervix	–	–	Unhelpful	Asymptomatic → moderate mucopurulent discharge
C. trachomatis infection	Cervix	–	–	Unhelpful	Asymptomatic → moderate mucopurulent discharge

FIG 25.1 Anatomy of sexually transmitted disease

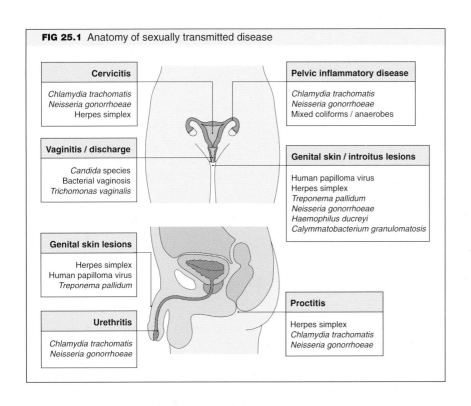

Cervicitis

Chlamydia trachomatis
Neisseria gonorrhoeae
Herpes simplex

Pelvic inflammatory disease

Chlamydia trachomatis
Neisseria gonorrhoeae
Mixed coliforms / anaerobes

Vaginitis / discharge

Candida species
Bacterial vaginosis
Trichomonas vaginalis

Genital skin / introitus lesions

Human papilloma virus
Herpes simplex
Treponema pallidum
Neisseria gonorrhoeae
Haemophilus ducreyi
Calymmatobacterium granulomatosis

Genital skin lesions

Herpes simplex
Human papilloma virus
Treponema pallidum

Urethritis

Chlamydia trachomatis
Neisseria gonorrhoeae

Proctitis

Herpes simplex
Chlamydia trachomatis
Neisseria gonorrhoeae

Case study 2

A 19 year old male presents to his GP with a 2 day history of urethral discharge and severe pain on passing urine. He has no history of previous genitourinary problems and is normally fit and healthy. On examination, he is apyrexial; there is a creamy discharge from his urethra, with slight reddening of the surrounding glans penis, but otherwise his genitals appear normal.

Questions

1. If you are his GP, what would you want to know in his history?

2. What is your differential diagnosis?

3. What would your immediate management be?

   He is referred to the local genitourinary medicine clinic where a Gram stain of the urethral discharge shows intracellular Gram-negative diplococci (i.e. cocci in pairs).

4. What is your diagnosis and management?

   The urethral discharge is subsequently reported as positive for *Chlamydia trachomatis*, and a 7 day course of doxycycline is commenced.

5. How common is a mixed infection like this?

   His regular partner is rather reluctant to attend the clinic because she feels well and has no discharge.

6. What is the likelihood of her being infected?

7. What would your management be?

   Five days later, she ends up back in the department complaining of a vaginal discharge that she didn't have before her 'treatment' (her inverted commas!).

8. What is your explanation?

Answers

1. The most important thing is to find out whether he is sexually active. He has a regular partner, his girlfriend, and denies any other sexual contact within the last 12 months. She takes the contraceptive pill — they do not use condoms.

2. This includes urethritis caused by *Neisseria gonorrhoeae* and *Chlamydia trachomatis*, as well as 'non-specific urethritis' — i.e. of unknown cause. Although gonococcal infection is frequently associated with this amount of discharge and pain, in practice a diagnosis could only be made following investigation.

3. The best plan would be to refer him immediately to the genitourinary medicine clinic. They have more experience with STDs, better facilities for diagnosing gonococcal and other infections and are much better placed for 'contact tracing' when appropriate.

4. This confirms the diagnosis of urethritis caused by *Neisseria gonorrhoeae*. Penicillin and tetracyclines are no longer appropriate because of bacterial resistance; he is given a single dose of 'ciprofloxacin' 500 mg and sent home. Efforts are made to contact his girlfriend.

5. It is rather difficult to obtain accurate figures, but the majority of males infected with *Neisseria gonorrhoeae* will probably have a co-existent infection with *Chlamydia trachomatis* as well. Although it is not invariable, the presence of one STD should always raise suspicion that there may be others present too.

6. *Neisseria gonorrhoeae* (and *Chlamydia trachomatis*) cause endocervicitis in the female which is *frequently asymptomatic*. If, as he has said, she is his only recent sexual contact, then she must be the source of his infection; if he is not disclosing another sexual contact from whom he acquired infection, she should still be investigated as he may well have transmitted the disease to her by now, the efficiency of male to female transmission of *Neisseria gonorrhoeae* being approximately 50–90% per sexual contact (as opposed to the approximately 20% risk of female to male transmission).

7. As her partner has evidence of both gonococcal and chlamydial infection, it would be reasonable to treat her without waiting for the results of specimens sent to the laboratory, particularly given her initial reluctance to attend the clinic. To eliminate the potential problem of compliance, she is given a single dose of azithromycin immediately, an antibiotic with an extremely long half-life that is active against both *N. gonorrhoeae* and *C. trachomatis*. However, she should be screened for both agents and possibly other STDs as well (such as infection with *Trichomonas vaginalis* and syphilis). She too, denies any recent sexual contact other than with her boyfriend, so that no further contact tracing is possible.

8. It is important to examine her properly. An endocervicitis would suggest a relapse or reacquisition of either gonococcal or chlamydial infection. However, a discharge that originates in the vagina itself would be new — most likely vaginal *Candida* overgrowth or bacterial vaginosis secondary to antibiotic therapy.

26 Obstetric and neonatal infections

Both the pregnant woman and the newborn infant are to some extent immunocompromised. Most infections in pregnancy are not more common (an exception is urinary tract infection) but are more likely to be severe or reactivate (**Table 26.1**). Primary infection in the mother induces IgM antibodies, but these do not pass the placenta to the fetus. Infection may result in fetal death and spontaneous abortion or **congenital** infection and associated malformations. The baby may also acquire infection around the time of birth (**perinatal** infection) or after birth (**postnatal** infection). Infections diagnosed in the first 3 months after birth are termed **neonatal** infections.

Prenatal / congenital infections

Most congenital infections (**Table 26.2**) follow primary maternal infection, but reactivation of CMV in pregnancy can lead to infection of the fetus. Many of the organisms responsible for congenital infections may also cause spontaneous abortion. Typically, most foetal infections are associated with mild or subclinical infections in the mother.

Diagnosis depends on clinical suspicion, contact history enhanced by serology of maternal blood. Confirmation may be made, via cordocentesis, by serology or PCR of fetal blood. First-trimester primary rubella infection caries such a high risk to the fetus of subsequent congenital rubella syndrome, that termination is usually advised if spontaneous abortion does not occur. Rubella infection after the fourth month does not pose a significant risk.

Perinatal infections

Most of the perinatal pathogens (**Table 26.3**) arise from the birth canal or blood. Some bacteria silently colonise the maternal genital and gastrointestinal tracts until ascending infection produces severe and disseminated disease in the baby. Such infections are more common when there has been premature rupture of membranes. **Early-onset** infection in the neonate (within the first week of life) usually presents as a severe septicaemia, whereas late-onset disease often presents as meningitis.

Other organisms are genital pathogens that may be acquired during delivery and generally cause localised rather then systemic infections. Eye infection in the newborn is known as **ophthalmia neonatorum**.

Postnatal infections

Infection acquired after birth may be associated with cross-infection from babies, their mothers and attendant staff in nurseries and neonatal intensive care units (**Fig. 26.1**). Staphylococcal infections are usually minor but may present as the 'scalded skin' syndrome. **Gastroenteritis** (bacterial or viral) can be life-threatening in low-birth-weight babies.

Diagnosis and management of neonatal infections

TORCH is an acronym for a screen for infections that are associated with neonatal disease. It stands for Toxoplasma, Rubella, Cytomegalovirus and Herpes simplex. It is a useful *aide memoire* but is by no means all-inclusive. Diagnosis of these infections is mainly serological, although the herpesviruses can be grown from infected sites. If confirmed then treatment (not available for rubella) should be given if symptomatic or, in the case of toxoplasma infections, even if asymptomatic to prevent long-term sequelae.

Chlamydial infections are detected by immunofluorescence or ELISA and treated with topical antibiotics.

With suspected covert bacterial infection, blood cultures and CSF must be cultured promptly together with swabs of superficial sites (e.g. umbilicus, ear and rectum). Urgent antibacterial treatment should then be started.

Risk factors for group B streptococcal disease can be identified and pregnant women screened for carriage of the organism in the vagina and rectum. Antibiotic prophylaxis is given to at-risk mothers during labour and to the baby after birth. Some viruses, e.g. HIV, may be transmitted by breast-feeding, which should be avoided.

Scrupulous attention to **aseptic techniques** and other infection control procedures is essential in the care of neonates.

Puerperal infections (postnatal infections in the mother)

Puerperal sepsis, caused by group A streptococci, is now uncommon since the introduction of hand washing by attendants and associated procedures.

Other organisms associated with puerperal infections include anaerobes and coliforms that may be introduced during instrumentation, especially septic abortions. The risk of infection is also increased if products of conception are retained in the uterus. Blood cultures and carefully taken high vaginal swabs should be sent and empirical antibiotic treatment started.

Staph. aureus may cause **breast abscesses** in the mother a week or so after birth.

TABLE 26.1

Effects of pregnancy on infection

More severe	May reactivate
Urinary tract infections	Cytomegalovirus (CMV)
Candida vulvovaginitis	Herpes simplex virus
Influenza	Epstein–Barr virus
Chicken pox (pneumonia)	Polyomavirus (BK, JC)
Viral hepatitis	
Poliomyelitis	
Malaria	
Listeriosis	
Coccidioidomycosis	

TABLE 26.3

Perinatal infections

Organism	Clinical features	Route of infection
Group B haemolytic streptococci	Meningitis, septicaemia	Ascending or during delivery
Esch. coli *Listeria monocytogenes*		
N. gonorrhoeae *Chlamydia trachomatis* Papillomavirus	Conjunctivitis Conjunctivitis, pneumonia Laryngeal warts	During delivery
Herpes simplex virus	Skin lesions, disseminated infection	Maternal blood at delivery
Hepatitis B virus HIV	Generalised infection	

TABLE 26.2

Congenital infections

Organism	Clinical features	Laboratory diagnosis	Preventative strategy
Rubella	Microcephaly, cataracts, deafness, heart defects, hepatosplenomegaly	Rubella IgM in cord blood Virus isolation (throat, urine)	Vaccination in childhood Screening in pregnancy
Cytomegalovirus	Deafness, mental retardation	CMV IgM in cord blood Virus isolation (throat, urine)	No current vaccine
Varicella-zoster	Skin, CNS and musculoskeletal abnormalities	Isolation of virus from vesicles, VZV IgM or rise in IgG	Anti-varicella-zoster immunoglobulin (for infections late in pregnancy)
Herpes simplex	Limb deformities, disseminated infection	Virus isolation	Caesarian section Prophylactic acyclovir
Hepatitis B	Hepatitis	Surface antigen in cord blood / PCR	Screening in pregnancy HBV immunoglobulin Vaccination of neonate
HIV	Failure to thrive, oral thrush, lymphadenopathy, hepatomegaly, childhood AIDS	HIV PCR as maternal antibody persists for up to 18 months	Screening in pregnancy Prophylactic antiretroviral therapy
Treponema pallidum	Lesions in skin, bones, teeth and cartilage Hepatosplenomegaly, lymphadenopathy	*T. pallidum* IgM in fetus	Screening in pregnancy Treatment of mother (early pregnancy)
Toxoplasma gondii	Microcephaly, eye lesions, Hepatosplenomegaly, jaundice	Toxoplasma IgM in cord blood	Selected screening in pregnancy Avoidance of primary infection Treatment of infection in pregnancy
Listeria monocytogenes	Septicaemia, meningitis, granulomas	Bacterial culture	None
Parvovirus	Anaemia, ascites, hepatosplenomegaly (hydrops fetalis)	Parvovirus IgM/PCR in cord blood	None

FIG 26.1 Routes of fetal and neonatal infection

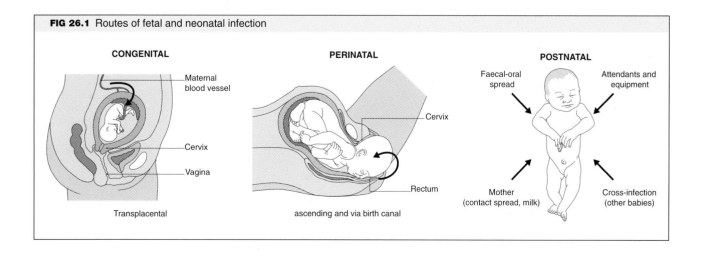

CONGENITAL

Maternal blood vessel

Cervix

Vagina

Transplacental

PERINATAL

Cervix

Rectum

ascending and via birth canal

POSTNATAL

Faecal-oral spread

Attendants and equipment

Mother (contact spread, milk)

Cross-infection (other babies)

27 Infections of bone, joints and muscle

Infections of bone and joint may arise from a number of sources (**Fig. 27.1**). Predisposing factors include:

- age — infections are commoner in neonates and the elderly
- pre-existing local pathology, e.g. trauma, tumours, sickle cell disease
- distant sites of infection, e.g. skin, chest, urine
- prosthetic material
- disorders of immunity, e.g. steroid or cytotoxic therapy.

The following clinical features may be present:

- fever (often with systemic illness)
- pain
- swelling
- erythema
- raised white cell count
- acute phase response ($\uparrow$ plasma viscosity and C-reactive protein).

Infections of bone — osteomyelitis

Infections may be classified as acute or chronic. The most frequent sites of infection are the lower limbs and the humerus.

In **acute osteomyelitis**, X-rays may not show an abnormality at presentation, but computerised tomography (CT) or white-cell scans can be helpful.

Systemic features are less common in **chronic osteomyelitis**, though local signs such as **sinus formation** may be present. **Periosteal reaction**, cysts **or sequestra** (dead bone within a cavity) may be seen on X-ray (**Fig. 27.2**). Blood cultures should always be taken and may be positive in about 50% of cases. Surgical material should be obtained for urgent microscopy and culture, particularly in chronic infections to guide long-term therapy.

Treatment may require both surgical drainage (which is usually essential in chronic cases) and antibiotic therapy. The choice of antibiotics should ideally be governed by culture results (see **Table 27.1**), but empirical therapy should include an anti-staphylococcal agent. Acute infections generally require 3–6 weeks therapy, but in chronic cases treatment should continue for several months with close monitoring of response. The parenteral route should be used for at least the first week and preferably longer.

Infections of joints — arthritis

Septic arthritis (Table 27.1) Most bacterial joint infections follow haematogenous spread and lead to **septic arthritis** with **joint effusions**, most commonly in the knee or hip. Chronic infections may develop, particularly with mycobacteria or fungi.

Reactive arthritis (Table 27.2) The sterile arthritis caused by an immune response to an infection is termed post-infectious or reactive arthritis. In many cases this follows infection with enteric pathogens and is associated with the HLA B27. In viral infections, e.g. rubella, multiple joints are often involved, especially the hands, wrists, knees, ankles and elbows, and the arthropathy 'flits' from one joint to another.

Investigation and management X-rays show distension of the joint capsule and soft-tissue swelling — destructive changes are only seen in cases which present late. These findings are not diagnostic of infection, and inflammatory conditions (e.g. rheumatoid arthritis and gout) need to be considered. Blood cultures should be taken and joint fluid aspirated. In bacterial infections about 50% of aspirates show bacteria in the Gram stain and 90% are positive on culture. Patients thought to have arthritis associated with gonococci or following gastrointestinal infections should have appropriate additional specimens taken. When tuberculosis is suspected synovial biopsies should be taken. Serology is used to determine viral infection.

Acute bacterial arthritis requires 2–3 weeks antibiotic treatment, initially by the i.v. route. Open **surgical drainage** may also be necessary.

Prosthetic joint infections have an incidence of < 1% following hip or knee replacement but are very difficult to diagnose and treat. Most infections are probably acquired at operation and often present months later. Coagulase-negative staphylococci are common pathogens and form a polysaccharide matrix, which binds the organisms to the prosthesis. Microbiological diagnosis requires careful culture of multiple operative specimens to distinguish pathogens from contaminant skin flora. Treatment usually requires complete removal of the joint and associated cement.

Infections of muscle

Acute bacterial cellulitis caused by Group A β-haemolytic streptococci may involve underlying fascia and muscles. Gangrene may follow trauma or infection with mixed organisms, including streptococci, anaerobes and coliforms. Both potentially fatal infections require prompt antibiotic therapy and full surgical debridement. **Viral myositis** produces self-limiting muscle pain and may be caused by coxsackieviruses, mumps or influenza. **Parasitic infections** include *Trypanosoma cruzii* (Chagas' disease) which may destroy cardiac muscle, *Taenia solium* which produces calcified muscle cysts, and *Trichinella spiralis* which causes fever and muscle pains.

TABLE 27.1

Pathogens of bone and joints and their treatment

Pathogen	Osteomyelitis		Septic arthritis	Empirical Treatment[a]
	Acute	Chronic		
Staph. aureus	✓✓	✓✓	✓✓	Flucloxacillin
Streptococci	✓	✓	✓	Penicillin
Enterobacteriaceae		✓	R	
Pseudomonas spp.		✓	R	
Anaerobes		✓	R	Metronidazole
H. influenzae	R		R	Ceftriaxone
M. tuberculosis		✓	✓	Izoniazid, rifampicin & pyrazinamide
Coag-neg staphylococci			✓	Vancomycin
N. gonorrhoeae			R	Penicillin
Brucella spp.		R	R	Tetracycline
Borrelia burgdorferi			R	Tetracycline
Viruses (see Table 27.2; antigen may be found with some viruses, but rarely true infection)			✓	
Fungi (*Sporothrix schenckii*)		R	R	Amphotericin B

✓✓ most common; ✓ less common; R rare
[a]Specific choice depends on susceptibility data

FIG 27.1 Sources of infection of bone, joint and muscle

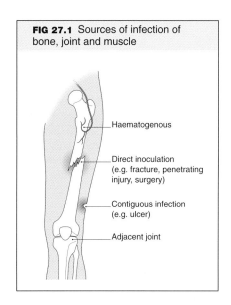

Haematogenous

Direct inoculation (e.g. fracture, penetrating injury, surgery)

Contiguous infection (e.g. ulcer)

Adjacent joint

TABLE 27.2

Causes of reactive arthritis

Strep. pyogenes
Salmonella
Shigella
Campylobacter
Yersinia
Borrelia burgdorferi (Lyme disease)
Chlamydia trachomatis
Mycoplasma pneumoniae
Rubella
B19
Hepatitis B virus
Ross River virus
Alphaviruses
Other viruses rarely

FIG 27.2 X-ray showing chronic ostemyelitis of the tibia

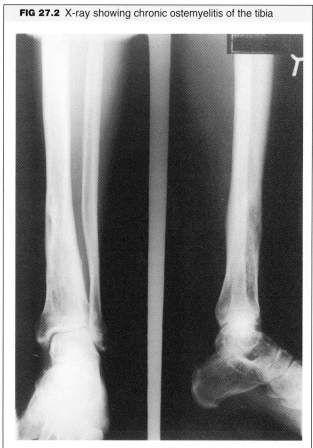

28

Septicaemia

Septicaemia is a clinical term describing signs of infection associated with micro-organisms in the blood stream. The term **bacteraemia** simply refers to the presence of bacteria in the blood, sometimes transiently, with or without symptoms. Septicaemia carries a high mortality and must be recognised, investigated and treated promptly.

The **risk factors** associated with septicaemia are shown in **Table 28.1**. The incidence of many community-acquired infections has changed little in recent years. In hospital-acquired infections the increasing use of invasive procedures, immunosuppressive therapy and broad-spectrum antimicrobials has lead to an increase in the proportion of Gram-positive isolates, especially coagulase-negative staphylococci and enterococci. **Fig. 28.1** shows the organisms isolated in a large teaching hospital laboratory.

The clinical features often include:

- fever, sometimes with rigors
- tachycardia
- hypotension
- confusion or agitation
- evidence of a focus of infection.

In severe cases the patient may present with circulatory collapse (**shock**) and the temperature may be paradoxically low. Acute infections are traditionally associated with Gram-negative bacteria but cannot be distinguished clinically from Gram-positive septicaemia. A careful history and examination may reveal the **source of infection** and help predict the likely organism (**Table 28.2**). Even in an emergency situation it is vital to collect at least one set of **blood cultures** (and preferably any other cultures) before antimicrobial treatment is started (see **Table 28.3**).

Blood cultures are generally incubated for 5–7 days but often become positive within the first 48 h. The first report is the **Gram stain** of the cultures that may allow a provisional early identification — possible coliforms, staphylococci, streptococci, etc. This information may help to identify the source of infection in the absence of clinical clues. The isolation of Gram-negative bacteria from blood suggests a urinary (or gastrointestinal) source; staphylococci might suggest a wound infection, abscess or osteomyelitis. The specific identification may give further help with the diagnosis: e.g. the *Streptococcus milleri* group is associated with abscess formation or infective endocarditis.

Careful interpretation of the **significance** of positive blood cultures is important. Skin organisms such as coagulase-negative staphylococci and diphtheroid bacilli often represent **contamination** but may be significant in line infections and prosthetic valve endocarditis. Further blood cultures taken from peripheral veins or through intravascular lines together with a careful review of the clinical findings (including other cultures) may allow a clearer assessment of significance. Such interpretations require close liaison between the microbiologist and clinician.

Positive cultures from blood (and other sites) also guide **antimicrobial therapy**. General suggestions for empiric therapy are given in **Table 28.2**. When **susceptibilities** are available, antimicrobial therapy is always reviewed and modified as required.

Blood cultures may be negative in septicaemic patients because:

- the patient has received antimicrobial therapy
- the bacteraemia is intermittent
- the patient has circulating bacterial toxins rather than viable organisms
- the media used are not optimal for fastidious organisms

Some organisms (e.g. pneumococci and meningococci) may be detected in blood (and other body fluids) by **non-cultural techniques** such as **antigen detection** or PCR. Techniques for detection of circulating toxins are not currently available for routine use.

Gram-negative septicaemia is most commonly associated with coliforms but may be caused by meningococci. **Endotoxin** released from Gram-negative bacteria leads to tissue damage mediated by cytokines such as interleukins and tumour necrosis factor. Current research into these mechanisms may identify agents that could be used to inhibit tissue damage. Severe disease may also accompany Gram-positive septicaemia, particularly *Staphylococcus aureus* and β-haemolytic streptococci, especially Group A (*Streptococcus pyogenes*).

The management of septicaemia requires more than appropriate antimicrobial therapy. The patient's general condition requires **close monitoring** with particular regard to cardiovascular, respiratory and renal function. Many patients will require fluid replacement, and the more severe cases may well require supportive management in an intensive care unit. The typical **complications** of severe septicaemia include:

- acute renal failure
- respiratory failure — acute respiratory distress syndrome (ARDS)
- haematological failure — disseminated intravascular coagulation (DIC).

Prevention of some cases of septicaemia is possible, particularly in the hospital setting. Successful interventions include:

- appropriate use of antimicrobial prophylaxis
- strict attention to aseptic technique and care of indwelling devices
- prompt diagnosis and treatment of infective sources.

TABLE 28.1

Septicaemia — examples of risk factors

Factor	Examples
Extremes of age	Neonates
Underlying disease	Diabetes
	Malignancy
	Immunosuppression
Septic focus	Urinary tract infection
	Respiratory tract infection
	Localised abscess
Surgery	Release of gastrointestinal flora
Broken skin	Traumatic or surgical wounds
	Burns
	Leg ulcers, bed sores
Invasive devices	Intravascular lines
	Urinary catheters
	Endotracheal tubes
	Prosthetic implants
Highly invasive pathogen	*Salmonella typhi*
	Neisseria meningitidis
	Streptococcus pyogenes

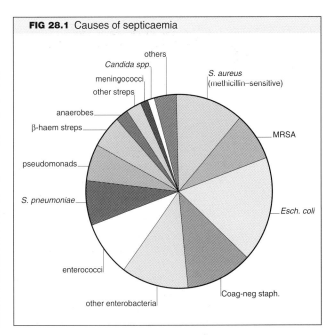

FIG 28.1 Causes of septicaemia

TABLE 28.2

Organisms in blood cultures — clinical associations and treatment

Organism	Associated with	Empirical antimicrobials[a]
Gram-negative		
Coliforms (*E. coli*, *Klebsiella* spp., etc)	Urinary tract infections	Gentamicin
	Gastrointestinal tract	
	Neutropenic sepsis	Gentamicin + piperacillin
Pseudomonas aeruginosa	Urinary tract	Gentamicin
	Respiratory tract (ventilated patients)	
Salmonella spp.	Enteric fever	Ciprofloxacin
	Invasive infections at extremes of age	
Neisseria meningitidis	Septicaemia	Benzylpenicillin
	Meningitis	
Haemophilus influenzae	Meningitis	Ceftriaxone
	Skin, bone and joint infections	
Gram-positive		
Staphylococcus aureus	Wounds and other broken skin sites	Flucloxacillin
	Intravascular line sites	(vancomycin for MRSA)
	Septic arthritis or osteomyelitis	
	Infective endocarditis	
Coagulase-negative staph.	Colonised intravascular lines	Vancomycin
	Infective endocarditis	
Streptococcus pneumoniae	Pneumonia	Benzylpenicillin (ceftriaxone
	Meningitis	for resistant strains)
Streptococcus pyogenes	Cellulitis	Benzylpenicillin
Group B streptococci	Obstetric and neonatal infections	
Enterococcus spp.	Colonised intravascular lines	Ampicillin
	Infective endocarditis	
Listeria monocytogenes	Meningoencephalitis	Ampicillin
Anaerobes		
Bacteroides spp.	Gastrointestinal tract	Metronidazole
Clostridium spp.	Female genital tract	
	Gangrene	
Fungi		
Candida spp.	Colonisation of intravascular line	Amphotericin
	Immunocompromised host	

[a]Examples only are given; specific choices depend on patient factors and local susceptibilities and prescribing policies — some patients may require alternatives or combination treatment

TABLE 28.3

Principles of blood culture technique[a]

- Disinfect hands using alcohol hand rub
- Identify suitable venepuncture site and/or intravascular line
- Disinfect patient's skin (e.g. using 70% alcohol) and allow to dry
- Prepare blood culture bottles (disinfecting tops of bottles if required)
- Collect blood sample (typically 20 ml from adults, 1–5 ml from children) without touching venepuncture site; use a different venepuncture for each blood culture set
- Inoculate blood culture bottles (typically aerobic and anaerobic set) — if other blood tests are required, always inoculate blood culture bottles before filling other specimen bottles, to avoid contamination
- Complete request form with full clinical details including site of sample (vein or intravascular line)
- Transport cultures rapidly to laboratory or place in incubator

[a]Specific details vary — check local hospital information

Case study 3

A 70 year old lady is admitted to hospital having suffered a 'stroke'. On admission she is comatosed, and it is noticed that she is incontinent of urine and has a bladder catheter inserted. She does not regain consciousness over the next week, during which period she has an i.v. infusion. On admission she is noticed to be febrile, temperature 38.0°C, but this subsides. On day 5 she is again febrile and has a temperature of 38.5°C. By day 7 her temperature has fallen but she is hypotensive and has poor urinary output.

Questions

1. How would you investigate the cause of fever?

2. A catheter specimen of urine (CSU) is taken and reveals white cells and over 10^5 bacteria per ml of mixed flora. How would you interpret this?

3. Results of examination and further investigation show:

    — Chest is clear except for crepitations at both bases.
    — Suprapubic specimen of urine shows white cells and over 10^5 E. coli/ml.
    — Blood cultures grow a 'coliform' in one bottle. What is the diagnosis?

4. How would you manage this case?

5. Is the urinary tract the only possible source of the bacteraemia?

6. What is the pathogenesis of the hypotension?

Answers

1. Fever may result from infectious and non-infectious aetiology. Strokes themselves may provoke fever — the likely reason for the initial fever. Common sites of infection in such patients are the lungs and urinary tract. The chest should be examined and a chest X-ray taken if appropriate. Samples of urine and blood should be taken for microscopy and culture.

2. Catheter specimens of urine are easily contaminated; this is borne out in this case by the mixed flora. The presence of leucocytes occurs with the trauma and irritation caused by the catheter. Notwithstanding, this does not rule out bladder infection.

3. The diagnosis is an *E. coli* urinary tract infection and septicaemia.

4. This is a 'grey' area in view of the patient's age and underlying condition. If her prognosis is generally good, then she would be managed 'aggressively' with removal of the urinary catheter, i.v. antibiotic therapy and management for shock.

5. Another possible source of infection in this patient is infection through her i.v. catheter, particularly if the site of entry is inflamed. This would necessitate removal of the catheter, and culture of the tip may confirm the clinical suspicion.

   In clinically significant bacteraemia, the urinary tract is the source in about 30%, the respiratory tract in about 15%, the gastrointestinal in 10%, biliary tract 10% and intravascular catheters 5%. *E. coli* is the commonest organism found if the source is urinary, gastrointestinal or biliary tracts; pneumococci and *S. aureus* are the commonest from a lung source; coagulase-negative staphylococci from intravascular catheters.

6. The pathogenesis of bacteraemic shock is complex. Some of the recognised pathways are shown in Case Study 3, Figure, p. 121.

29 Acquired immunodeficiency syndrome (AIDS)

AIDS is the commonest cause of death in young adults in many parts of the world. The major burden of infection is in Africa, S.E. Asia and India, and S. America where heterosexual transmission predominates and the number of cases in men and women are approximately equal. In Europe and North America, homosexual transmission has been responsible for the majority of cases. Apart from transmission by sex, transfer has also occurred by blood and blood products, including injectable drug use, and vertically from mother to child.

The viruses There are two viruses — Human Immunodeficiency Virus (HIV) type 1 and HIV-2 — which are accepted causes of AIDS. Structurally, these viruses are identical (**Fig. 29.1**). They are retroviruses, so-called because they encode an enzyme, **reverse transcriptase** (RT), that makes a DNA copy of genomic RNA when it infects cells; this is 'backwards' (Greek *retro*) to the classic RNA from DNA. The replication cycle of HIV-1 is shown in **Fig. 29.2**.

The viruses undergo rapid evolution, with quasispecies being produced as the RT enzyme makes mistakes in copying the original genome. These are grouped as strains or **clades**, with HIV-1B being the virus that was first recognised in the USA.

HIV disease and pathogenesis HIV infects T lymphocytes and macrophages. These cells express receptors for the virus, CD4 (and others such as CCR5). Early infection takes place predominantly in the lymph nodes, although CD4-positive cells in tissues such as the brain and gut are also infected. This initial infection elicits a vigorous immune response which is detectable as anti-HIV antibody after 4–8 weeks. In many cases this primary illness (or 'seroconversion illness') is manifest as a glandular fever-like illness 2–12 weeks after initial infection. Uncommonly, infection is aborted at this stage, but in the majority there follows a long incubation period with continued viral replication (over 10 billion new viruses per day) accompanied by a large turnover of immune cells. This period lasts months and years, with increasing lymph node activity which can be eventually detected clinically as a **persistent generalised lymphadenopathy** (PGL). As the destruction of immune cells becomes greater than new production, AIDS develops.

AIDS AIDS is symptomatic HIV infection. It is a clinical diagnosis made with the presence of a number of 'AIDS-defining illnesses', usually with detectable anti-HIV antibody. These illnesses are, with few exceptions, **'opportunistic' infections** and tumours. There are several international definitions of AIDS, but the most common examples of infections and tumours found are given in **Table 29.1**.

Diagnosis of HIV infection The presence of antibodies to structural proteins, particularly gp120, is detected by ELISA or Western blot analysis to confirm infection with HIV. There is, however, a **window period** (up to 3 months is generally accepted as the time period for reliability of a negative response) where the antibody response is not detectable by current serological assays. In neonates, the presence of maternal antibody makes serological diagnosis difficult for up to 18 months. If infection is considered to be likely then PCR detection of viral genome is the test of choice. Quantitative PCR to determine **viral load** is also the preferred method of monitoring progression and treatment of disease (CD4 count is a common alternative).

Management of HIV disease In the early stages there is treatment of HIV itself, but with the onset of immunosuppression, there is also the management and prophylaxis of opportunistic infections and tumours.

HIV is best treated with a combination of antiretroviral drugs (**Fig. 29.2**). Treatment is probably best instituted early in infection when the balance between the host immune system and virus is still in favour of the former. All the currently available drugs have serious side-effects, and treatment needs to be adjusted to minimise these.

Drug therapy is complicated when opportunistic infections arise, as there is a high risk of adverse drug interactions. Management is best undertaken in specialist centres, as this area of antimicrobial drug development is the most active and new drugs are emerging rapidly and being used before licensing,

A vaccine for HIV would be ideal but is beset by the rapid evolution of the virus.

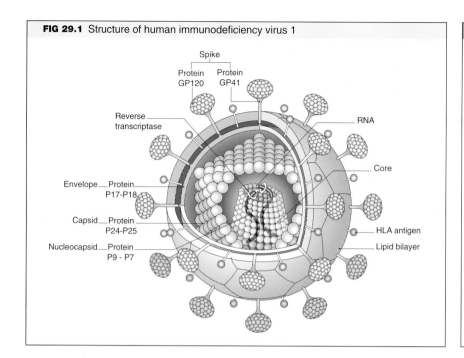

FIG 29.1 Structure of human immunodeficiency virus 1

Spike
Protein GP120
Protein GP41

Reverse transcriptase

RNA

Core

Envelope — Protein P17-P18

Capsid — Protein P24-P25

Nucleocapsid — Protein P9 - P7

HLA antigen

Lipid bilayer

TABLE 29.1

Common diseases in AIDS

Infections
- Candidiasis (oral, oesophageal, tracheal, lung)
- Cytomegalovirus (retinitis and elsewhere)
- *Pneumocystis carinii* pneumonia
- Atypical mycobacterial infections
- Persistent diarrhoea (*Cryptosporidia, Isospora, Encephalitozoon* spp., etc.)
- Cryptococcus infections (meningitis, pneumonia)
- Herpes simplex infections (disseminated, gastrointestinal, pneumonia)
- Encephalopathy (HIV, toxoplasmosis)
- Tuberculosis (disseminated)
- Coccidiodomycosis
- Salmonellosis
- Recurrent bacterial pneumonia
- Severe wasting

Tumours
- Kaposi's sarcoma (skin, disseminated)
- Burkitt's and other lymphomas
- Invasive cervical cancer
- Oral hairy leukoplakia

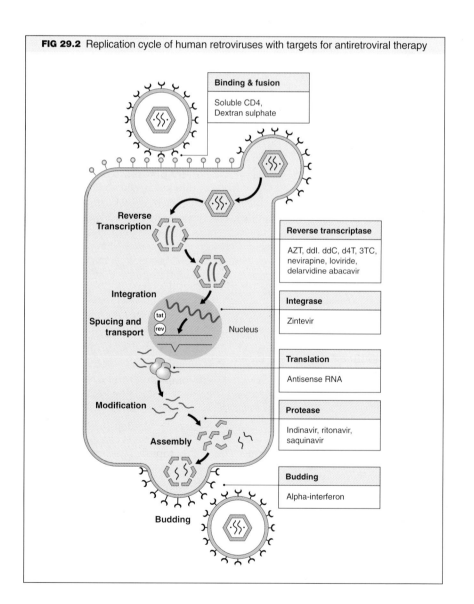

FIG 29.2 Replication cycle of human retroviruses with targets for antiretroviral therapy

Binding & fusion
Soluble CD4, Dextran sulphate

Reverse Transcription

Reverse transcriptase
AZT, ddI. ddC, d4T, 3TC, nevirapine, loviride, delarvidine abacavir

Integration

Integrase
Zintevir

Spucing and transport

tat
rev

Nucleus

Translation
Antisense RNA

Modification

Protease
Indinavir, ritonavir, saquinavir

Assembly

Budding
Alpha-interferon

Budding

Infectious mononucleosis and other systemic infections

There are infections that most commonly manifest as fever and/or a non-localised infection. Many infections can present in this way but have a predilection for a particular organ system and are described elsewhere.

Infectious mononucleosis This is also called glandular fever because of the presence of generalised lymphadenopathy. It is most commonly caused by primary infection with **Epstein–Barr virus** (EBV), a herpesvirus (**Fig. 30.1** and **Table 30.1**). Sore throat, tonsillar enlargement and palatal petechiae also occur; with the potential complications of splenomegaly, hepatitis and autoimmune haemolytic anaemia. Large numbers of atypical monocytes in a blood film, the presence of cold agglutinins and a **heterophil antibody** response to horse or sheep erythrocytes, which causes a positive Paul–Bunnell or Monospot test, is also typical. Confirmation of EBV infection is made by specific serology. Treatment is supportive.

EBV is an aetiological agent in a number of other diseases (**Table 30.2**).

Other common infectious causes of generalised lymphadenopathy, with or without fever, are cytomegalovirus and *Toxoplasma gondii*. The former is generally acquired during childhood via saliva, although other body fluids may also contain virus. Infection is more typically silent but, as with other herpesvirus infections, reactivation occurs. It is a common cause of fever in post-transplant patients, and of retinitis and pneumonia in AIDS. Primary infection during pregnancy or at term is particularly problematic, as congenital infection may result. 5% of these will be symptomatic at birth, with jaundice, eye, brain and other abnormalities. These have a poor prognosis. The others are asymptomatic at birth, but a minority of these patients will have hearing impairment and other defects later in childhood. Diagnosis depends on detecting the virus in urine, blood or saliva and/or serologically. Complications require treatment.

Toxoplasmosis is a zoonosis, with cats as the predominant source of infection for humans. The commonest presentation is of a transient febrile illness, often with lymphadenopathy; but intrauterine infection may cause stillbirth or congenital abnormalities, and infection in the immunocompromised may result in cerebral infection with characteristic multiple calcified lesions seen on X-ray. The dye test which utilises patient serum to kill viable toxoplasma in vitro is being replaced by specific ELISA assays for

diagnosis. Serious illness, and those occurring in pregnancy, require treatment, with drugs such as pyrimethamine, spiramycin and atovaquone, often in combination.

Q fever and other rickettsial infections

Coxiella burnetii infection is a zoonosis from sheep which presents as a non-specific fever but may progress to an atypical pneumonia and/or endocarditis. Diagnosis is based on the detection of complement-fixing antibody to phase 1 antigen (acute Q fever) or to phase 1 and phase 2 antigens (chronic Q fever). Treatment is with a prolonged course of tetracycline or erythromycin.

Other rickettsial infections have arthropod vectors (ticks, mites and fleas) and cause flu-like illnesses with or without a petechial rash: typhus, Rocky Mountain spotted fever, Mediterranean spotted fever, rickettsial pox and trench fever being the best recognised. Serological tests are used to confirm the diagnosis, and treatment is usually with tetracyclines.

Mycobacterial infections Tuberculosis is most commonly caused by *M. tuberculosis*, and less often by the related *M. bovis*, *M. microti* and *M. africanum*. Clinically, there is primary disease which most commonly occurs in the lung with a Ghon focus of tubercle bacilli and hilar lymphadenopathy, the so-called **primary complex**. Post-primary tuberculosis is manifest as tuberculomata, granulomatous lesions with caseous 'cheesy' necrosis, in the lung and elsewhere. Diagnosis is based on microscopy of infected material with Ziehl–Neelsen staining, and culture which may take several weeks. Treatment is with a combination of drugs to reduce drug resistance and enhance therapy. The **tuberculin** test, intradermal inoculation of purified (tuberculous) protein derivative (PPD), is also a useful diagnostic and screening test, although it does not distinguish between active and old infection and previous BCG vaccination.

Other mycobacteria also cause disease (**Table 30.3**).

Plague This is a disease still present in many parts of the world. Caused by *Yersinia pestis*, it presents as a bite from an infected rodent with local tender lymphadenopathy ('buboes') and fever. Multisystem involvement can occur with high mortality. Organisms can be identified from lymph nodes or sputum (in pneumonic plague) and should be treated with streptomycin and/or tetracycline.

TABLE 30.1

Human herpesviruses

Designation	Common name	Diseases
Human herpesvirus 1 (HHV-1)	Herpes simplex type 1 (HSV-1)	Oral, skin and genital ulcers, encephalitis, disseminated infection in newborn and immunocompromised
Human herpesvirus 2 (HHV-2)	Herpes simplex (HSV-2)	Same as HSV-1 but more common cause of genital ulcers
Human herpesvirus 3 (HHV-3)	Varicella-zoster virus (VZV)	Chickenpox, herpes zoster, disseminated zoster in immunocompromised
Human herpesvirus 4 (HHV-4)	Epstein–Barr virus (EBV)	Glandular fever, Burkitt's lymphoma & other lymphoproliferative conditions, nasopharyngeal cancer, oral hairy leukoplakia, chronic interstitial pneumonitis in AIDS
Human herpesvirus 5 (HHV-5)	Cytomegalovirus (CMV)	Glandular fever, congenital syndrome, retinitis & disseminated infection in AIDS
Human herpesvirus 6 (HHV-6)	(HHV-6)	Roseola infantum
Human herpesvirus 7 (HHV-7)	(HHV-7)	None yet
Human herpesvirus 8 (HHV-8)	Kaposi's sarcoma (KSHV)	Probably Kaposi's sarcoma

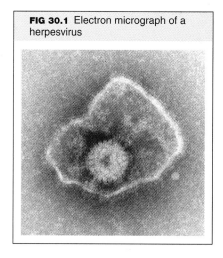

FIG 30.1 Electron micrograph of a herpesvirus

TABLE 30.2

Diseases associated with Epstein–Barr virus infection

Disease	Diagnostic viral markers	Comments
Infectious mononucleosis	Monospot & heterophil antibody positive Raised VCA IgG & IgM Raised EA-D IgG	Peaks of incidence in pre-school children and young adults
Silent primary infection	Monospot & heterophil antibody positive Raised VCA IgM & IgG Raised EA-R IgG EA-D IgG negative	
Burkitt's lymphoma	Raised VCA IgG VCA IgM & IgA negative Raised EBNA IgG Raised EA-R IgG	Predominantly occurs in equatorial Africa. Malarial infection appears to be a co-factor
Nasopharyngeal carcinoma	Raised VCA & EA IgA & IgG Raised EA-D & EBNA IgG EA-R negative	Commonest in S. E. Asia, North & Central Africa
X-linked lymphoproliferative syndrome	Raised VCA & EA IgG Low EBNA IgG	Sporadic cases also occur in females
Post-transplant lymphoproliferative syndrome	Raised VCA & EA IgG	May result in widespread lymphoma
Oral hairy leukoplakia	Not useful clinically	AIDS
Chronic interstitial pneumonitis	VCA IgM positive	AIDS
Chronic EBV infection	Positive Monospot Raised VCA & EA-D IgG Absent EBNA 1 IgG	Causes chronic lethargy

EA, early antigen; D, diffuse; R, restricted; EBNA, Epstein–Barr virus-associated nuclear antigen; VCA, viral capsid antigen

TABLE 30.3

Manifestations of non-tuberculosis mycobacterial infections

Disease	Agent
Pulmonary infection	M. avium complex M. kansasii M. malmoense M. xenopi
Lymphadenopathy	M. avium complex M. scrofulaceum
Swimming pool granuloma	M. marinum
Buruli ulcer	M. ulcerans
Skin abscesses	M. chelonae M. fortuitum M. terrae
Disseminated disease	M. avium complex M. chelonae
Tuberculoid leprosy	M. leprae
Lepromatous leprosy	M. leprae

31 Infections of the immunocompromised host

An **immunocompromised** or **immunodeficient** person is lacking in some aspects of innate and/or adaptive immunity. This may be due to a **primary** deficiency or, far more commonly, a deficiency **secondary** to some other condition. If induced deliberately through medical intervention, during tumour therapy or after transplant, for example, the person is described as being **immunosuppressed**. Whatever the route, the net result is that the immunocompromised individual becomes susceptible to:

- infection with a range of **opportunistic** pathogens, such as the commensal flora *in addition to* more conventional agents
- infections that may be more severe than in a 'normal' host.

Although it is important to recognise when a patient is immunocompromised, in some ways this very broad term is unhelpful because it does not allow an estimate of the most likely causes of infection. This depends on how the patient's condition affects each limb of the immune system, as shown in **Table 31.1**, which in turn controls the most likely pathogens (**Table 31.2**). It should be noted that immunity varies throughout life and not just in 'disease' states.

The details are beyond the scope of this book, but chronic renal failure is given as an example:

- Chronic renal failure leads to a moderate but broad suppression of adaptive immunity and phagocytic function so that the number of infections is increased slightly and agents such as *Legionella, Salmonella* and *Listeria* can be problematic. However, the chief concern arises from breaching the skin for CAPD or haemodialysis, and staphylococcal infections are therefore frequent (**Table 31.1 and 31.2**).
- If a renal transplant is undertaken, the immediate potential infective problems are those relating to major surgery: pneumonia as a result of intubation and artificial ventilation; line-related sepsis with intensive care support; wound infection secondary to surgery; and serious infection relating to manipulation of the urinary tract.
- Long-term post-transplant, infective problems are determined by the degree of immunosuppression required to prevent transplant rejection, with opportunistic pathogens reflecting a decrease in cellular immunity (**Tables 31.1 and 31.2**).

It is important to have this background information because it allows the development of protocols for the prevention, investigation and treatment of infections in immunocompromised patients, which present a number of particular problems for clinical management:

- Antibiotic prophylaxis or immunisation may reduce the frequency of infection, e.g. penicillin and pneumococcal vaccine to decrease pneumococcal infections after splenectomy. In highly susceptible bone marrow transplant patients, exposure to fungal spores may be diminished by treating their air supply with high-efficiency particulate air (HEPA) filters. Patients should be made aware of the infections to which they are particularly susceptible so that they can reduce their risk of exposure (e.g. by more careful food preparation to decrease the potential for *Salmonella* and *Campylobacter* infection) and obtain medical advice if they are exposed (e.g. exposure to varicella-zoster virus by contact with a case of chickenpox).
- Accurate diagnosis of infection can be difficult because of an unusual presentation: the disease may be more extensive than normal and the characteristic symptoms/signs may be lacking without an immune response. In cases where there is little inflammation, the **focus of infection** may be unknown, making it difficult to guess the most probable pathogens.
- Antibiotic prophylaxis may make culture from patient samples difficult within the laboratory. Because these patients may have had so many antibiotics in the past, infection with antibiotic-resistant bacteria is more likely.
- Opportunistic pathogens may require unusual diagnostic methods within the laboratory (and also unusual treatments). Serology as a diagnostic method is unhelpful because it presumes an effective immune response within the patient. Laboratory culture results may be difficult to interpret, as the commensal flora, which are usually regarded as **contaminants** that were inadvertently picked up when the sample was taken, may be opportunistic pathogens in the immunocompromised host.
- Treatment may have to/ be more aggressive than for the same pathogen in a host with a normal immune system and may need to be extended for longer periods, possibly even for life.

TABLE 31.1

Defects in immunity in specific conditions

Haematological malignancy
- ↓↓ neutrophil and lymphocyte numbers
- ↓ antibody production

Neonates
- open umbilicus
- incompetent blood–brain barrier
- ↓ antibody levels
- ↓ complement
- ↓ antibody response to polysaccharide
- ↓ neutrophil function

Elderly
- atrophy/dryness of skin/mucous membranes
- ↓ cellular immunity associated with altered lymphocyte subsets (mature v immature; naïve v memory; Th1 v Th2)

Malnutrition
- thinning skin/mucous membranes
- ↓ lysozyme production
- ↓ cellular immunity
- ↓ phagocyte function
- ↓ complement
- ↓ antibody including IgA
- ↓ cytokine production

Diabetes
- skin breaches (injections, vascular disease and neuropathy)
- ↓ neutrophil chemotaxis
- ↓ phagocyte adherence
- ↓ phagocytosis (if ↑↑ glucose)
- ↑ Candida urine colonisation if ↑ urinary glucose

Chronic renal failure
- skin breaches (CAPD, haemodialysis)
- ↓ lymphocyte numbers
- ↓ cytokines (⇒ ↓ number, accumulation and chemotaxis of phagocytes)

Alcoholism
- ↑ risk aspiration stomach contents
- ↓ cough reflexes
- ↑ risk trauma
- lifestyle
- ↓ complement
- ↓ T cell function

Steroids
- ↓ neutrophil/monocyte accumulation chemotaxis
- ↓ lymphocyte numbers, especially T cells

Cytotoxics
- ↓↓ neutrophil, monocyte and lymphocyte numbers

Cyclosporin A
- ↓ T_4 cell function

TABLE 31.2

Defects in immunity and infection

	Innate immunity			Adaptive immunity	
Physical defences	Complement	Phagocytes		Humoral immunity	Cellular immunity
Main class of micro-organism					
Bacterial	Bacterial	Bacterial/fungal		Bacterial	Intracellular agents
Specific pathogens					
Skin					
S. aureus	Neisseria	S. aureus		Enteroviruses	All viruses esp.
Streptococcus	H. influenzae	S. pneumoniae		Rotavirus	herpes viruses
	S. pneumoniae	Gram-negatives			adenoviruses
	S. aureus			S. aureus	
Respiratory					
Respiratory viruses		Aspergillus		S. pneumoniae	Mycobacterium
S. pneumoniae		Candida		H. influenzae	Listeria
H. influenzae				Salmonella	Salmonella
M. catarrhalis				Campylobacter	Legionella
					Nocardia
Gastrointestinal					
Salmonella				Giardia lamblia	Candida
Campylobacter					Aspergillus
Gram-negatives					Cryptococcus
Anaerobes					Pneumocystis
Urinary					
E. coli					Toxoplasma
Gram-negatives					Cryptosporidium
					Strongyloides
Genital					
Anaerobes (bacterial vaginosis)					
Candida					

32 Zoonoses

Zoonoses are infections transmitted from animals to man. They are caused by various bacteria, viruses, fungi, protozoa and helminths. Animals serve as natural reservoirs for the micro-organisms and do not usually show signs of disease. Domestic and farm animals are the predominant reservoirs of disease in Europe, and wild animals in the tropics.

Many zoonoses are occupational diseases affecting farmers, vets, animal breeders, slaughterhouse and laboratory workers.

Zoonoses result from:

- **direct contact** with animals, their excreta and saliva
- **indirect contact** though food and water contaminated with excreta or saliva
- **arthropod vectors** through the bite of an insect, louse or tick.

Within these groups, zoonoses may be further classified by the mode of transmission, intermediate host and whether infection is part of the life cycle:

- **cyclozoonoses:** require more than one vertebrate host, but no invertebrate host for transmission (e.g. tapeworm)
- **metazoonoses:** infectious organisms must multiply or develop in an invertebrate host before transmission to a vertebrate host is possible (e.g. plague and schistosomiasis)
- **saprozoonoses:** development outside of a vertebrate host is required, such as on vegetation or in soil (e.g. *Toxocara* spp.).

Direction of transmission Although zoonoses are usually considered to be diseases transmitted from animals to man, they may also be transmitted from man to animals, or in either direction. These are termed:

- **anthropozoonoses:** transmission from animals to man
- **zooanthropozoonoses:** transmission from man to animals
- **amphixenoses:** infection maintained in both man and animals, and may be naturally transmitted in either direction.

Impact of zoonoses Zoonoses represent some of the most prevalent and serious infections world-wide. Examples of common zoonoses are shown in **Table 32.1**. In the United Kingdom zoonotic infections are uncommon, and many that were once endemic have declined or been eradicated in recent years (e.g. rabies, anthrax and brucellosis). However, the 'new' zoonoses of campylobacter enteritis, *Escherichia coli* (VTEC strains) and cryptosporidiosis are being reported with increasing frequency (**Table 32.2**). Changes in farming practices, reflecting the increased demands of the consumer, have undoubtedly contributed to the greater incidence of such infections.

Emerging zoonoses In recent years, many of the newly recognised infectious diseases of man have been traced to animal reservoirs (e.g. campylobacter enteritis, cryptosporidiosis, Lassa fever). It therefore seems probable that future human pathogens will be identified as zoonotic in origin rather than through the appearance of a completely new pathogenic agent.

Factors influencing such events might include microbial changes at the molecular level, such as acquisition of virulence factors, and modification of the immunological status of individuals and populations. The impact of AIDS has seen the emergence of many 'new' opportunistic infections as well as the increased prevalence of other recognised pathogens. Social and ecological conditions that influence population growth and movement, farming and dietary habits, and the environment may also play a significant role.

Diagnosis As with other microbial infections, zoonotic diseases can be diagnosed by standard laboratory techniques of culture, microscopy, immunological and molecular analysis. When performing such investigations it is important to determine the occupation and hobbies of a patient, as a history of animal contact may indicate a zoonotic infection.

TABLE 32.2

Incidence of zoonoses in the United Kingdom

Disease	Organism	Incidence per annum
Brucellosis	*Brucella abortus*	<10
Leptospirosis	*Leptospira interrogans*	50
Lyme disease	*Borrelia burgdorferi*	<10
Salmonellosis	*Salmonella*	30 000
Campylobacter	*Campylobacter*	50 000 (rising)
Haemorrhagic colitis and haemolytic uraemic syndrome	*Escherichia coli* (VTEC)	1500 (rising)
Psittacosis	*Chlamydia psittaci*	600
Q fever	*Coxiella burnetii*	200 (underestimated)
Orf	Orf virus	50
Toxoplasmosis	*Toxoplasma gondii*	500 congenital infections
Cryptosporidiosis	*Cryptosporidium parvum*	5000
Ringworm	Tinea (dermatophyte fungi)	Unknown but common

TABLE 32.1

Examples of common zoonoses

Disease	Organism	Animal reservoir	Mode of transmission	Symptoms	Distribution
Bacteria					
Brucellosis	*Brucella*	Cattle, goats, pigs	Birth products, food and dairy produce	PUO, lymphadenopathy, splenomegaly, nausea,weight loss	World-wide
Salmonellosis	*Salmonella*	Most animals	Food and dairy produce	Acute diarrhoea, abdominal pain, low-grade fever	World-wide
Campylobacteriosis	*Campylobacter*	Most animals, notably chickens	Food and dairy produce	Actue, diarrhoea, pain and fever	World-wide
Verotoxigenic Escherichia coli (VTEC)	*Escherichia coli*	Cattle	Food and dairy produce	Acute diarrhoea, renal failure	World-wide
Bubonic plague ('Black Death')	*Yersinia pestis*	Wild rodents (especially rats)	Flea bite	Fever, swollen, tender lymph nodes (buboes), pneumonia, black skin necrosis	South-western USA, Africa and Asia
Leptospirosis (Weil's disease)	*Leptospira interrogans*	Rats	Urine contamination of wound or eye	Myalgia, malaise, chills, fever, renal and hepatic failure	World-wide
Anthrax	*Bacillus anthracis*	Most mammals	Animal hides	Cutaneous pustules, fever, malaise, headache, sepsis, pneumonia ('woolsorter's disease')	World-wide
	Pasteurella multocida	Oral cavity of most mammals	Saliva from animal bite (especially dog or cat)	Inflammation at bite or scratch, abscess and cellulitis	World-wide
Lyme disease	*Borrelia burgdorferi*	Most animals, (especially deer and rodents)	Tick bite	Rash, flu-like symptoms, arthritis	World-wide
Psittacosis	*Chlamydia psittaci*	Birds	Inhalation of bird respiratory secretions	Atypical pneumonia (flu-like, dry cough)	World-wide
Q-Fever (Query fever)	*Coxiella burnetii*	Wild and domestic animals, especially sheep and cattle	Birth products, urine, faeces and milk	Atypical pneumonia, febrile illness, subacute endocarditis	World-wide
Endemic typhus	*Rickettsia typhi*	Rodents	Louse bite	Fever, flu-like symptoms, rash, meningoencephalitis, coma	World-wide
Viruses					
Orf	Parapoxvirus	Sheep and goats	Direct animal contact	Large painful nodules usually on hands	World-wide
Rabies	Rhabdovirus	All mammals	Saliva from bite, scratch or abrasion	Severe pain at bite site, hydrophobia, muscle spasms, laryngospasm, extreme excitability: high mortality rate	World-wide (some exceptions)
Ebola	Filovirus	Unknown: possibly monkeys	Person to person	Fever, headache, malaise, chest discomfort, diarrhoea and vomiting: fatality rate is 50–90%.	Northern Zaire and Southern Sudan
Lassa fever	Arenavirus	Rodents	Rat excreta contamination of skin abrasions, food, water, or airborne	Fever, haemorrhaging, renal failure	West Africa
Yellow fever	Flavivirus	Monkeys	*Aedes* mosquito bite	Fever, jaundice, haemorrhaging	Central and South America and Africa
Fungi					
Taenia ('ringworm')	*Microsporum canis*	Dogs and cats	Direct contact with animal	Skin, hair, nail infections	World-wide
Cryptococcosis and histoplasmosis	*Cryptococcus neoformans* and *Histoplasma capsulatum*	Possibly birds	Inhalation of spores from bird droppings	Pneumonia and meningitis	World-wide
Protozoa and helminths					
Toxoplasmosis	*Toxoplasma gondii*	All mammals (cats are definitive host)	Ingestion of cat faeces or contaminated meat	Mild (flu-like), severe (multi-organ infection)	World-wide
African trypanosomiasis	*Trypanosoma*	Domestic cattle and pigs	Tsetse fly bite	General febrile illness followed by CNS invasion and coma	East and West Africa
American trypanosomiasis		Domestic and wild animals	Triatomid bug excreta, contamination of bite or eye	Fever, lymphadenopathy, hepatosplenomegaly, cardiac and CNS involvement	Mexico, Central and South America
Cryptosporidiosis	*Cryptosporidiosis parvum*	Most mammals	Contaminated water and food	Mild to severe diarrhoea	World-wide
Toxocariasis	*Toxocara canis* and *cati*	Dogs (*canis*) and cats (*cati*)	Ingestion of faeces	Fever, cough, hepatomegaly, splenomegaly and lymphadenopathy; granuloma of the retina	World-wide
Tapeworm: cysticercosis	*Taenia saginata* and *solium*	Cattle (*saginata*) and pigs (*solium*)	Ingestion of contaminated meat	Abdominal pain, diarrhoea and weight loss: cysticerci in muscles	World-wide (rare in developed countries)

Case study 4

A group of thirty primary school children visited a local farm during which they came into close contact with various animals and were allowed to handle lambs. Packed lunches, prepared at the homes of the children, were eaten during the visit. Over the next 3–5 days eight of the children developed severe diarrhoea without vomiting that persisted for 1–3 weeks. Several family members of the affected children also subsequently developed the same symptoms.

The local Environmental Health Department was notified, and an investigation into the possible source of the outbreak was instigated. This revealed that no children from other classes at the school were absent with similar symptoms nor were there any reports of similar symptoms in the communities where the children lived. The farm visit was the only common feature shared by all the infected children.

Questions

1. What questions would help identify or eliminate sources of the outbreak?

   Faecal specimens were also taken from the children and sent to the microbiology laboratory for examination.

2. What tests would you request the laboratory to undertake on the specimens, and why are investigations for viral causes not indicated here?

   Culture results for enteric pathogens were all negative. However, microscopy on stained preparations of faecal smears showed numerous spherical parasite oocysts.

3. What is the likely identity of the organism seen on microscopy?

4. How did infection arise in the children, and why were some family members who did not go on the farm visit infected?

5. What is the term applied to human infections acquired from animals?

6. What other pathogens causing diarrhoea can be acquired from contact with animals?

Answers

1. Pathogenic organisms causing diarrhoea are transmitted by food, water, animals and humans. Outbreaks of such disease can usually be traced to a common source. In this instance children from other classes were not affected, eliminating the school meals or local water supply as the source. No cases occurred in neighbouring homes of those affected, further indicating that the source was not water-borne. The common feature was the recent visit by the class to a local farm.

2. Culture and microscopy for common bacterial (e.g. *Campylobacter*, *Salmonella*, *Shigella*, *Escherichia coli*) and protozoal (e.g. *Cryptosporidium parvum*, *Giardia lamblia*, *Entamoeba histolytica*) causes of diarrhoea. The outbreak is unlikely to be due to a viral cause, as the time for onset of symptoms was several days and no vomiting was involved.

3. *Cryptosporidium parvum*, an intestinal parasite causing cryptosporidiosis.

4. Cryptosporidiosis is transmitted by ingestion of oocysts that are shed in the faeces (faecal-oral route). The disease also occurs in animals, and in this instance the probable source was the lambs handled by the children (oocysts were then either ingested directly off the hands or on the food when the packed lunches were eaten). Cryptosporidiosis can also be transmitted from person to person, giving rise to family outbreaks of infection.

5. Zoonoses.

6. Bacteria: *Escherichia coli*, *Salmonella* and *Campylobacter*. Protozoa: *Giardia lamblia* and possibly *Entamoeba histolytica*.

33 Malaria

Malaria is an infection of liver and red blood cells caused by protozoan parasites of the genus *Plasmodium*. Malaria is one of the most serious health problems facing humanity today, affecting four hundred million people world-wide and causing 2 million deaths each year. Four species infect man: *P. falciparum* (the most common and dangerous), *P. malariae*, *P. ovale* and *P. vivax*.

Life cycle

Malaria is spread by the bite of an infected *Anopheles* mosquito. Only females of the species bite humans and transmit the disease. The parasite has a complex life cycle involving sexual reproduction in the mosquito and asexual reproduction in liver parenchymal cells and erythrocytes (red blood cells) in humans (**Fig. 33.1**):

1. *In the mosquito*:
   (a) Male and female **gametocytes** from an infected human are ingested when mosquito feeds.
   (b) **Gametocytes** undergo sexual reproduction in stomach to form an **oocyst** containing **sporozoites**.
   (c) Oocyst penetrates the gut wall and the sporozoites enter salivary glands.
   (d) Sporozoites infect human when mosquito next feeds.

2. *In humans*:
   (e) Sporozoites enter the blood and infect parenchymal liver cells.
   (f) Asexual reproduction (**schizogony**) forms **schizonts** in which thousands of **merozoites** develop.
   (g) Merozoites rupture from the liver schizonts and enter erythrocytes.
   (h) Ring-form trophozoites, then sporozoites and finally merozoites develop.
   (i) Merozoites rupture from the cells to invade other erythrocytes.
   (j) Some merozoites form gametocytes that infect the female mosquito at next feed and continue life cycle.

In *P. ovale* and *P. vivax* infection, some sporozoites remain dormant as **hypnozoites** in the parenchymal cells, only starting the process of schizogony months or years later.

Epidemiology In spite of intensive control measures, malaria remains widely distributed in the tropics and subtropics of Africa, Asia and Latin America (**Fig. 33.2**). *P. falciparum* and *P. vivax* account for 95% of all malaria cases, and 80% of these occur in tropical Africa.

- *P. falciparum* and *P. malariae* are the predominant species in the tropics.
- *P. vivax* is common in the tropics, subtropics and some temperate regions.
- *P. ovale* is common in West Africa.

Clinical features The repeated rounds of erythrocyte invasion and rupture release toxins that cause bouts of high fever. Classic symptoms include:

- cycles of shaking chills followed by fever and profuse sweating
- anaemia and jaundice due to erythrocyte destruction
- dark pigmented urine ('blackwater fever') from erythrocyte destruction
- liver and spleen enlargement and renal failure.

The time between these fever episodes can be characteristic of the infecting *Plasmodium* species (**Table 33.1**). With *P. falciparum* this is every 36–48 h (**malignant tertian malaria**) compared with 72 h for *P. malariae* (**quartan malaria**). The cycle is also 48 h for *P. vivax* but the symptoms are less severe (**benign tertian malaria**).

Cerebral involvement is a serious consequence of falciparum malaria. The high levels of parasitaemia lead to the schizont-containing erythrocytes blocking brain capillaries. The resulting hypoxia causes confusion, coma and death.

The dormant liver hypnozoites formed in ovale and vivax malaria can result in relapse many years after the initial infection.

Diagnosis Malaria should be suspected in any case of fever associated with travel to endemic areas. Diagnosis is made by clinical symptoms and microscopic examination of blood to identify the erythrocytic forms. This permits the differentiation of *Plasmodium* species which is vital in the correct choice of treatment.

Treatment Malaria can normally be cured by antimalarial drugs (**Table 33.1**). Chloroquine is the drug of choice, although resistance by *P. falciparum* has restricted its effectiveness in many parts of the world. Alternative drugs are quinine, mefloquine and the combination of sulfadoxine plus pyrimethamine. However, resistance to these agents is also being reported. Primaquine is included in ovale and vivax malaria to destroy the liver hypnozoites.

Prevention Vaccines are being developed but are not yet available against malaria. Travellers to endemic areas must protect themselves from infection and seek expert advice about antimalarial prophylaxis before embarking. The regimen for drug prophylaxis depends on whether resistance is present in the area. Examples include chloroquine, fansidar, pyrimethamine plus dapsone and chloroquine plus proguanil. Preventing mosquito bites by covering limbs, using insect repellents and sleeping under mosquito nets is also essential. Stagnant water, the breeding ground of mosquitoes, should also be avoided.

TABLE 33.1

Human malaria infections

Species	Distribution	Incubation period (liver cycle)	Duration of fever (erythrocytic cycle)	Clinical condition	Major complications	Treatment
P. falciparum	West, East and Central Africa, Middle East, Far East, South America	7–14 days	36–48 h	Malignant tertian malaria	Cerebral malaria, haemolytic anaemia ('blackwater fever'), jaundice, hypoglycaemia	Chloroquine, quinine, mefloquine, sulfadoxine and pyrimethamine
P. vivax	India, North and East Africa, South America, Far East	12–17 days (with relapse up to 3 years)	48 h	Benign tertian malaria	Relapse due to liver hypnozoites	Chloroquine with primaquine
P. malariae	Tropical Africa, India, Far East	13–40 days (with rare relapse)	72 h	Quartan malaria	Nephrotic syndrome	Chloroquine with primaquine
P. ovale	Tropical Africa	9–18 days (with relapse up to 20 years)	48 h	Ovale tertian malaria	Relapse due to liver hypnozoites	Chloroquine with primaquine

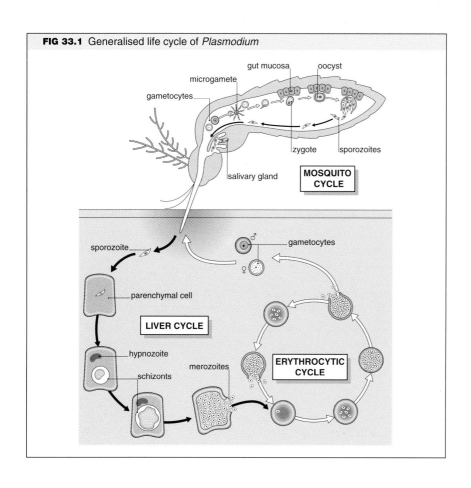

FIG 33.1 Generalised life cycle of *Plasmodium*

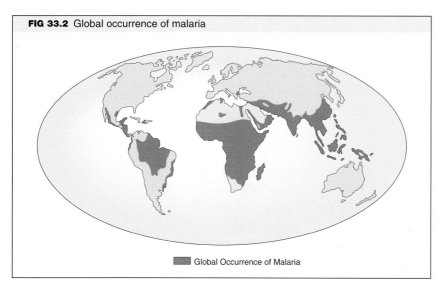

FIG 33.2 Global occurrence of malaria

Global Occurrence of Malaria

Case study 5

A 36 year old man visited his general practitioner after sudden onset of fever with chills, cough and myalgia. A week previously he had returned to England after a 6 month contract working as a civil engineer in Rwanda and Uganda. He told the doctor that he had returned from Africa the previous day and had not taken malaria prophylaxis.

Routine haematological tests performed in the surgery showed haemoglobin (Hb) 13.2 g/dL, white blood cell (WBC) count 3.0×10^9/L, platelets 100×10^9/L and erythrocyte sedimentation rate (ESR) 70 mm/h. Blood cultures, urine and faecal specimens were taken along with thick and thin blood films and sent to the laboratory.

Questions

1. What is the suspected diagnosis from this information?

2. What is the purpose of the laboratory investigations?

   Four days later the patient was admitted to hospital because of high fever, mental confusion, abdominal pain and dysuria. On examination his temperature was 39.7°C, pulse 112/min and BP 110/70 mmHg. Laboratory investigations showed Hb 11.0 g/dL, WBC 3.4×10^9/L, platelets 80×10^9/L, sodium 143 mmol/L, potassium 3.6 mmol/L, urea 8 mmol/L, creatinine 200 μmol/L. He remained drowsy and confused but with no neck stiffness and appeared slightly jaundiced. He described the pattern of fever and chills occurring approximately every 2 days.

   The blood, faecal and urine cultures were negative and no intestinal parasites were seen on microscopy. The blood films were also negative. Repeat thick blood films were prepared and sent for examination and antimalarial treatment started (quinine in this case).

3. What remains the suspected diagnosis?

4. Based on the cycle of the fever and chills what is the probable malaria type?

   The laboratory examination of the repeat thick blood films confirmed the diagnosis of malaria, identifying *Plasmodium falciparum* as the cause. However, the patient continued to deteriorate, becoming comatosed and hypotensive. Two days later he had a cardiac arrest from which he could not be resuscitated.

5. What two major complications associated with falciparum malaria are shown here?

6. What problems are associated with antimalarial chemotherapy?

7. Describe the preventive measures this patient should have used to avoid infection?

Answers

1. Malaria is the diagnosis that should be first considered, but typhoid and other infections should also be considered in anyone returning from the tropics with a fever.

2. Culture of blood, urine and faeces for bacterial pathogens (particularly typhoid); microscopy of faeces for intestinal parasites; staining of blood films to identify blood parasites (especially malaria).

3. Malaria, based on cycle of fever and chills, jaundice, falling haemoglobin. Thick blood films are preferred for malaria diagnosis. However, a negative result does not exclude the infection, as the level of erythrocyte infection can be very low and organisms may not be present in the blood film examined.

4. Malignant tertian malaria due to *Plasmodium falciparum* (approx. 48 h cycle of the fever).

5. Cerebral malaria and acute renal failure ('blackwater fever').

6. Drug resistance and dormant liver hypnozoites in *P. ovale* and *P. vivax* malaria that cause relapse many years after the initial infection. Treatment should be aimed at both hepatic and extrahepatic infection.

7. Malaria prophylaxis (which should be commenced a week before leaving home and continued for 4 weeks after returning) and avoiding mosquito bites (covering the body and sleeping under mosquito nets). Advice for the best current regime should be taken from specialist centres, as the susceptibility of parasites to specific drugs varies globally.

34 Other tropical infections

Tropical infections affect millions of people world-wide, causing considerable human suffering and economic hardship. Far from declining, the incidence of many tropical infections is increasing throughout the world. The impact of human immunodeficiency virus (HIV) and AIDS has seen the emergence of 'new' opportunistic pathogens as well as the increased prevalence of other recognised types. Climatic changes induced through global warming have aided the spread of many diseases, whilst starvation and the breakdown in sanitation that accompanies war has seen the re-emergence of others. In addition, the development of drug resistance has also dramatically influenced the ability to treat and control many diseases, notably parasitic infections.

Clinicians in the West will encounter tropical infections. The ease and speed with which the globe can be traversed by air travel and the quest for ever more exotic holiday destinations means patients can become infected and return home before symptoms have developed. Refugees and immigrants can also import infections into the country or acquire them on visits home.

Tropical infections may be broadly classified as those causing fever, diarrhoea and skin diseases. They are caused by a variety of bacteria, viruses and parasites as summarised in **Table 34.1**. More common examples are described below.

Fever

Malaria is the prime suspect in any patient presenting with fever after returning from a risk area (e.g. the tropics and subtropics of Africa, Asia and Latin America). A blood film examination for the parasite is an urgent investigation.

Typhoid and paratyphoid fevers are highly infectious bacterial causes and present as fever with abdominal discomfort or vague abdominal pains, rose spots on the trunk and splenomegaly. Infected persons may become asymptomatic excretors of the organism.

Tuberculosis (TB) in the United Kingdom is 30–200 times as common in immigrants as in the indigenous population. This is probably because of increased susceptibility to the infection and can take a form unfamiliar to doctors not educated in third-world countries. HIV infection greatly increases the risk of TB, and the AIDS pandemic has seen a resurgence of the disease.

Other causes of subacute or chronic imported fever include:

- *viruses:* viral hepatitis, Lassa fever, rabies
- *bacteria:* tick typhus, brucellosis, relapsing fever

- *parasites:* amoebic liver abscess, early schistosomiasis, visceral leishmaniasis, African and American trypanosomiasis.

Diarrhoea

Diarrhoea is a common complaint after foreign travel, and acute cases will be caused by food-poisoning organisms found also in the West (e.g. salmonella, shigella, campylobacter, enteric viruses). Tropical causes are likely to be protozoa or helminths. Infections are usually asymptomatic in the native population but can be severe when acquired by the non-indigenous visitor.

Bacteria Cholera causes severe diarrhoea that may be fatal because of extensive electrolyte and water depletion. It is endemic where standards of sanitation and hygiene are low. Up to 10% of the patient's body weight can be lost in a few hours through the 'rice-water stool' that arises from the infection.

Protozoa and helminths Amoebiasis and giardiasis are the commonest infective causes of chronic diarrhoea. Persistent eosinophilia implicates a worm infection, most commonly filariasis, schistosomiasis and occasionally strongyloidiasis. Other causes are:

- **ascariasis** (the large roundworm)—heavy infections may cause a variety of complications, including intestinal obstruction
- **trichuriasis** (whipworm)—chronic bloody diarrhoea, anaemia and rectal prolapse when very large numbers are present
- **hookworms**—can cause significant blood loss resulting in iron deficiency anaemia
- **tapeworms**—infections are common, but autoinfection by the pig tapeworm (cysticerosis) can be life-threatening.

Skin conditions

Ulcers are the most common skin lesions in the tropics. The cause is usually unknown, although Vincent's organisms (a fusiform and a spirochaete) and β-haemolytic streptococci are often isolated on culture. Mycobacteria, corynebacteria and the protozoan parasite *Leishmania* are also important causes.

Leprosy is caused by an acid-fast mycobacterium and spread by person-to-person contact. The condition is characterised by a variety of symptoms, but the most important is thickening of peripheral nerves leading to localised areas of anaesthesia in the affected tissues. Some ten million people are affected world-wide.

TABLE 34.1

Examples of tropical infections

Disease	Organism	Symptoms	Mode of transmission	Distribution	Treatment
Bacteria					
Cholera	*Vibrio cholera*	Copious watery diarrhoea ('rice-water stool')	Faecal-oral from contaminated water	World-wide: India, South-east Asia and South America	Fluid + electrolyte replacement; oral tetracycline
Bubonic plague ('Black Death')	*Yersinia pestis*	Fever, swollen lymph nodes ('buboes'), pneumonia, black skin necrosis	Rodent fleas	South-western USA, Africa and Asia	Streptomycin + tetracycline
Endemic typhus	*Rickettsia typhi*	Fever, flu-like symptoms, rash, meningoencephalitis, coma	Louse bite	World-wide	Tetracycline
Leprosy	*Mycobacterium leprae*	Lepromatous: (progressive) skin nodules, nerve involvement Tuberculoid: skin lesions (benign), severe nerve and tissue destruction	Person-to-person contact	Africa, India, South-east Asia and South America	Dapsone + rifampicin
Tropical ulcer	*Mycobacterium ulcerans*	Buruli ulcer: gross, necrotising ulceration of the skin	Unknown	Tropical areas in all continents	Clofazimine or rifampicin
Tuberculosis	*Mycobacterium tuberculosis*	Pulmonary: cough, chest pain, fever, dyspnoea, haemoptysis and weight loss Glandular involvement (in tropics) associated with HIV infection	Person to person through respiratory secretions; milk from infected cattle	World-wide	Ethambutol, isoniazid, rifampicin, pyrazinamide (in combination)
Typhoid and paratyphoid fever	*Salmonella typhi* and *paratyphi*	Fever and systemic infection from invasion of bloodstream	Faecal-oral	World-wide	Co-trimoxazole, ciprofloxacin, ceftriaxone

TABLE 34.1 *(cont'd)*

Examples of tropical infections

Disease	Organism	Symptoms	Mode of transmission	Distribution	Treatment
Viruses					
Rabies	Rhabdovirus	Severe pain at bite, hydrophobia, muscle spasms, laryngospasm, extreme excitability	Saliva via bite, scratch, or abrasion	World-wide (some exceptions)	None
Ebola	Filovirus	Fever, headache, malaise, chest discomfort, diarrhoea and vomiting	Person to person	Northern Zaire and southern Sudan	None
Lassa fever	Arenavirus	Fever, haemorrhage, renal failure	Rat excreta contamination of skin abrasions, food, water, or airborne	West Africa	None
Yellow fever	Flavivirus	Fever, jaundice, haemorrhage	*Aedes* mosquito	Central and South America and Africa	None
Protozoa					
Amoebiasis	*Entamoeba histolytica*	Bloody diarrhoea and occasionally liver infection	Faecal-oral via cysts in food and water	Common in tropics	Metronidazole, tinidazole
Balantidiasis	*Balantidium coli*	Mild to severe diarrhoea	Faecal-oral from cysts in food and water	Common in tropics	Tetracycline, iodoquinol
Malaria	*Plasmodium* species	Liver, blood and CNS infection	Mosquito	Africa, Asia and Latin America	Chloroquine, quinine, mefloquine, sulfadoxine + pyrimethamine, primaquine
African trypanosomiasis	*Trypanosoma gambiense* and *rhodesiense*	General febrile illness followed by CNS invasion	Tsetse fly	East and west Africa	Pentamidine, melarsoprol
American trypanosomiasis	*T. cruzii*	Fever, lymphadenopathy, hepatosplenomegaly, cardiac and CNS involvement	Triatomid bug	Mexico, Central and South America	Nifurtimox and benznidazole
Leishmaniasis	*Leishmania*	Skin sores (cutaneous) nose, mouth, palate destruction (mucocutaneous)	Sandfly	North Africa, India (cutaneous); Mexico, Central and South America (mucocutaneous)	Stibogluconate, meglumine antimonate, amphotericin B or pentamidine

TABLE 34.1 *(cont'd)*

Examples of tropical infections

Disease	Organism	Symptoms	Mode of transmission	Distribution	Treatment
Helminths					
Hookworms and Strongyloidiasis	*Ancylostoma duodenalis*, *Necator americanus* and *Strongyloides stercoralis*	Gut, lungs and heart infection; malnutrition, pneumonitis, anaemia	Larval infection through skin	Mediterranean, southern USA, Central and South America, Africa, Asia	Mebendazole, albendazole; thiabendazole, ivermectin (strongyloidiasis)
Ascariasis ('roundworm')	*Ascaris lumbricoides*	As for hookworms	Faecal-oral ingestion of eggs	Southern USA, Central and South America, Africa, Asia, Australia	Mebendazole or albendazole
Trichuris ('whipworm')	*Trichuris trichiura*	Gut infection, malnutrition	Faecal-oral ingestion of eggs	As for *Ascaris*	Albendazole or mebendazole
Bancroftian filariasis	*Wuchereria bancrofti*	Fever and lymphangitis leading to obstruction of the lymphatics	Mosquito	South America, Central Africa, Far East	Ivermectin or DEC
Onchocerciasis ('river blindness')	*Onchocerca volvulus*	Lymphadenopathy in groin and axilla, intradermal oedema and pachyderma, keratitis, retinochoroiditis	Blackfly	Central America, Central Africa and the Yemen	Ditto
Loaiasis ('eyeworm')	*Loa loa*	Migration of worm in eyelid, vitreous and anterior chamber	Mango fly	Central and West Africa	Ditto
Taeniasis (beef tapeworm)	*Taenia saginata*	Asymptomatic or abdominal pain, diarrhoea and weight loss	Ingestion of cysticerci in beef	World-wide	Praziquantil or niclosamide
Cysticercosis (pork tapeworm)	*Taenia solium*	Cysticercosis (pork tapeworm): larvae penetrate gut and form cysticerci in muscles	Ingestion of cysticerci in pork	South and Central America, China, Indonesia	Ditto
Schistosomiasis ('bilharzia')	*Schistosoma*	Liver and bladder (*S. haematobium*) or rectum (*S. mansoni, S. japonicum*)	Burrowing into skin of schistosome cercariae from aquatic snails	South America, West Indies, Africa, Middle East, Egypt, Far East	Praziquantel

35 Pyrexia of unknown origin

The majority of patients present with symptom/physical sign complexes compatible with only a few diseases, and they require little investigation. Other clinical presentations, such as **pyrexia** or **fever of unknown origin** (PUO or FUO), are more difficult because they have few signs and symptoms, so that the list of differential diagnoses is large and the need for investigation correspondingly greater. 'Classic' PUO has three features:

- an illness of more than 3 weeks' duration
- a temperature greater than 38.3°C (101°F) on several occasions
- no specific diagnosis after a week of hospital inpatient investigation.

With the changing pattern in hospital admissions, shorter inpatient times and more use of community and outpatient services, and also the development of a greater range of powerful diagnostic procedures, the third criterion may be replaced by a minimum set of investigations (**Table 35.1**) rather than a timed period in hospital. There are over two hundred reported diverse causes of PUO, which vary slightly according to age (**Fig. 35.1**). As the number of conditions that has to be considered is so large, some clinicians divide patients into further categories such as **neutropaenic PUO, nosocomial PUO** and **HIV- associated PUO**, to focus on particular causes and therefore streamline their investigation.

It is important to get a prompt diagnosis, as this may improve the prognosis for the patient through early treatment, and also prevent the risk of transmission to others in the case of communicable infections such as tuberculosis. Investigation is expensive both in time and resources, and it is equally important to ensure that the patient does indeed have a pyrexia and that it is not a **factitious** fever. Body temperature is normally higher in the evening than the morning, but some healthy individuals have an exaggerated circadian temperature rhythm. Others may invent physical diseases to gain medical attention (**Munchausen syndrome**), and an unexplained temperature is one means of doing this, either by manipulating the temperature recording device or even injection of contaminated materials.

Investigation Every case requires a comprehensive history, *careful* and *repeated* physical examination, as well as a range of diagnostic tests and procedures. History should include a thorough systems review with particular care concerning travel, occupational history and hobbies, pets and animal contact, drug prescriptions and other drug intake, familial diseases, previous illness and alcohol consumption.

A complete examination should include examination of the teeth, ears, fundoscopy and review of the skin in good light for faint rashes. This must be repeated at frequent intervals to spot important developing or fleeting physical signs. Temperature should be recorded methodically, although the great majority of patients never display the characteristic patterns of fever described in the textbooks.

Investigation may include: samples sent for laboratory testing; non-invasive tests such as diagnostic radiology and ultrasound and radionuclide scanning; skin testing, essentially the **tuberculin** test for infection with *Mycobacterium tuberculosis*; and invasive testing such as biopsy, endoscopy and surgical exploration. A possible minimum set of investigations is listed in **Table 35.1**; further investigation will depend upon what has already been done, and clues that may be obtained from the history and examination, working through all the possible differential diagnoses.

Causes Some well-recognised causes of PUO are given in **Table 35.2**. However, in the majority of cases, the cause is a familiar disease with an unusual presentation, rather than a rare disorder:

- Infections are the single most common cause of PUO, particularly in the young. They may be difficult to diagnose because the patient was on antibiotics when the sample was taken, because the site of infection is hidden or because the infectious agent is difficult or impossible to culture in the laboratory.
- Neoplasms are an important cause of PUO, particularly in the elderly. Certain tumours seem to cause pyrexia themselves, others may produce it because of necrosis or secondary infection.
- Collagen-vascular disease.
- Miscellaneous.
- Undiagnosed: this category is largely made up of patients who recovered from a benign **febrile** illness before a specific diagnosis was made.

Management There is no treatment for the clinical presentation of PUO itself; success lies in finding the cause of the PUO and then managing that condition.

TABLE 35.1

Possible minimum diagnostic evaluation for PUO

- Comprehensive history
- *Repeated* and *complete* physical examination
- Complete blood count, including differential and platelet count
- 'Routine' blood chemistry, including lactate dehydrogenase, bilirubin and liver enzymes
- Urinalysis, including microscopic examination
- Chest X-ray
- Erythrocyte sedimentation rate (ESR)
- Antinuclear antibodies
- Rheumatoid factor
- Angiotensin converting enzyme
- Multiple blood films (if any possibility of malaria)
- Blood cultures (3 sets) whilst *not receiving antibiotics*
- Cytomegalovirus IgM antibodies or virus detection in blood
- Heterophile antibody tests or EBV serology (children and young adults)
- Tuberculin skin test
- CT of abdomen/radionuclide scan
- HIV serology or virus detection assay
- Further evaluation of any abnormality detected by above

FIG 35.1 Causes of PUO at different ages

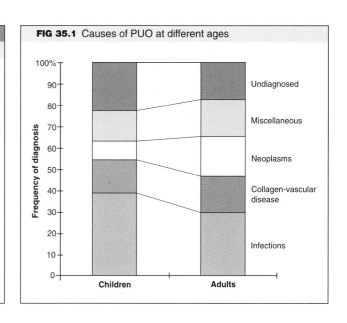

TABLE 35.2

Some causes of PUO

Infection	
Localised infection	Abscess: abdominal, dental, pelvic, intracranial
	Endocarditis and mycotic aneurysm, osteomyelitis, pyelonephritis, sinusitis, mastoiditis
Specific infections	
• Viral	Cytomegalovirus, Epstein–Barr virus, hepatitis viruses, HIV, parvovirus B19
• Bacterial	*Mycobacterium tuberculosis* (tuberculosis), *Brucellae abortus* or *melitensis* (brucellosis), *Legionella pneumophila* (Legionnaire's disease), *Bartonella henselae* (cat scratch fever), *Chlamydia psitta* (psittacosis), *Coxiella burnetti* (Q fever), *Salmonella typhi* (typhoid), *Campylobacter, Leptospira, Borrelia recurrentis* (relapsing fever) and *burgdorferi* (Lyme disease), *Treponema pallidum* (syphilis)
• Fungal	*Candida, Aspergillus, Cryptococcus neoformans, Histoplasma, Coccidioides, Blastomyces, Sporothrix*
• Parasitic	Malaria, giardiasis, toxocariasis, toxoplasmosis, trypanosomiasis, schistosomiasis, leishmaniasis
Neoplastic	Many tumours but especially lymphomas, leukaemias, renal-cell carcinoma and atrial myxoma
Collagen-vascular disease	Still's disease, rheumatoid arthritis, systemic lupus erythematosus (SLE), Reiter's syndrome, rheumatic fever, Felty's syndrome Various vasculitides
Miscellaneous	Haematoma, recurrent pulmonary embolism Drug fever, metal poisoning Crohn's disease, ulcerative colitis, sarcoidosis Familial fevers, cyclical neutropaenia
Undiagnosed	???

36 New and re-emerging infectious diseases

There has been considerable success in combating infection in the developed world over the last fifty years, through advances in nutrition and hygiene as well as the development of drugs and vaccines. The world-wide eradication of **smallpox** was a notable success, but 'new' infections are constantly being described (**Appendix 6**, p. 130), and there is always the problem of established infections becoming resistant to current therapies (**Table 36.1**). And there are few diseases that can have such a dramatic effect on human health as those that are caused by infection (**Fig. 36.1**).

New diseases

Viruses are potentially the most rapidly evolving of all infectious agents and therefore the greatest future threat. Bacteria may acquire or generate new virulence genes and become able to cause new infections. Alternatively the micro-organisms may not change but, because of changes in the environment that surrounds us, they may suddenly start to cause human disease.

- *Escherichia coli* 0157 and *Haemophilus influenzae* biogroup Aegyptius are probably 'new' pathogens.
- *Legionella pneumophila* (related to widespread airconditioning) and probably bovine spongiform encephalopathy/variant Creutzfeld–Jacob disease (probably related to changes in animal rendering) are pathogens resulting from changes in the environment.

Established diseases of unknown cause

When the aetiology of a disease is first discovered there may be a greater appreciation of its significance, although the disease itself is neither new nor the numbers necessarily increasing. A number of newly identified pathogens are listed below with the method of their detection, but there are likely to be many other diseases which may have an infectious aetiology, possibly even including conditions like sarcoidosis, multiple sclerosis and bipolar depression:

- *Borrelia burgdorferi*, *Campylobacter* spp. and *Helicobacter pylori* (laboratory culture)
- *Cryptosporidium* spp. and *Cyclospora* spp. (microscopy)
- *Tropheryma whippelii* and *Bartonella henselae* (molecular biology).

Re-emerging diseases

The **incidence** of many infections fluctuates with known **periodicity** over time — either due to changes in the physical environment, such as the peaks of food-borne illness associated with the warm summer months, or probably due to changes in levels of immunity within the population, such as the 9 yearly cycle of parvovirus infections. However, for some diseases, these changes may be unpredictable and dramatic. Pandemics of influenza virus infection, killing millions of people, have occurred in the past and may well do so again. Human *Salmonella* infections (**Fig. 36.2**) have varied considerably because of changing patterns of food consumption. The resurgence in cases of *Mycobacterium tuberculosis* infection in the USA, including cases with multiple-antibiotic resistance, results from running-down of public health facilities, immigration, and also HIV infection as it has increased the number of susceptible individuals who then form an increased reservoir of infection to be passed on to others.

The future?

As our civilisation develops, it is possible to appreciate a number of changes which benefit society but which may also be potential threats to world health from infectious disease, including:

- rapid, global transport, especially air travel, might allow a problem to be disseminated before it is recognised
- changes in food production — new methods may create new problems, but also, with the increasing industrialisation of production, problems with a single producer may affect vast numbers of people
- exploration and use of unknown, potentially threatening environments such as the rain forest (and, possibly, outer space)
- **xenotransplantation** and the risk of modifying animal diseases to infect humans
- increasing size and density of urban populations, and also an ever-increasing number of immunosuppressed individuals
- the effects of global warming.

It is clearly important that there should be sufficient infection **surveillance** in the population to recognise and to react quickly to any new threat; the American government and World Health Organisation have already set up groups specifically for this. There should be ongoing development of treatments so that they can be adapted to novel situations quickly and effectively.

TABLE 36.1

Emerging problems of drug resistance

Infectious agent	Resistance problem
Herpes simplex virus	Acyclovir
Human immunodeficiency virus	Zidovudine and others
Methicillin-resistant *Staphylococcus aureus* (MRSA)	β-lactams (and other antibiotics)
Vancomycin-resistant *S. aureus* (VISA or VRSA)	MRSA now also resistant to vancomycin
Penicillin-resistant *Streptococcus pneumoniae*	β-lactams (and other antibiotics)
Neisseria gonorrhoeae	Penicillin, tetracycline, quinolones
Glycopeptide-resistant *Enterococcus* spp. (GRE)	Multi-resistance including glycopeptides
Multi-drug-resistant *Mycobacterium tuberculosis* (MDR-TB)	Isoniazid, pyrazinamide, rifampicin and others
Gram-negatives with 'extended spectrum β-lactamases' (ESBL)	β-lactams (and other antibiotics)
Candida spp.	Fluconazole
Plasmodium spp.	Chloroquine
Scabies	Lindane

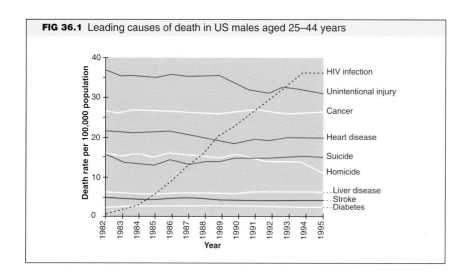

FIG 36.1 Leading causes of death in US males aged 25–44 years

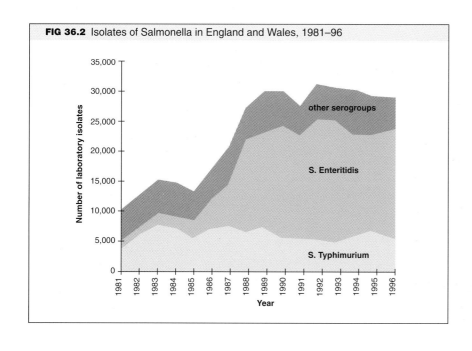

FIG 36.2 Isolates of Salmonella in England and Wales, 1981–96

Control of infectious disease

37 Principles of hospital infection control

Hospital infection increases patient morbidity, mortality, length of stay and treatment costs. It is estimated that about five thousand patients die as a result of hospital-acquired infection in Britain each year. Control of infection is therefore an essential element of hospital practice.

Definitions

Infections acquired by patients or staff in hospital are termed hospital-acquired or nosocomial (**Figs 37.1 and 37.2**). The **source** of infection may be other people (**cross-infection), the patient's own organisms (**endogenous infection) or via contaminated food, fluids equipment or the environment. In England the **prevalence** of hospital-acquired infection is approximately 10%, whereas the annual **incidence** is nearer 5%. The sources of hospital-acquired infections are shown in **Fig. 37.3**.

Control of hospital infection

Each hospital has an infection control officer (usually a consultant microbiologist) and infection control nurse(s) who together constitute the infection control team. This team advises on the prevention and control of hospital infection, utilising policies provided and updated by the hospital infection control committee. The team also monitors infection by **surveillance** — typically this involves tracking so-called **alert organisms** from sites such as wounds (e.g. *Staph. aureus* (including MRSA) and *Strep. pyogenes*), faeces (e.g. *Salmonella* spp. and *Clostridium difficile*) and respiratory tract (e.g. *Mycobacterium tuberculosis*). Another important function of the infection control team is **education** for all groups of staff to update them on new issues and improve compliance with policies.

The three principles of infection control are:

I: Exclude the source of infection Inanimate sources of infection can be identified and in many cases excluded from hospitals by ensuring the provision of:

- sterile instruments, dressings and intravenous fluids
- clean linen
- uncontaminated food and drink
- cleaned and disinfected or disposable equipment
- a safe and clean environment including water and air of appropriate quality
- clear policies for safe disposal of hospital waste.

Both patients and staff may act as a source of infection, so:

- Infected and colonised patients should be identified by adequate microbiological investigations and infections treated with appropriate antimicrobials.

- Staff should have health checks before employment and have necessary immunizations.
- Staff should report infections (e.g. diarrhoea) and needlestick injuries.

II: Prevent transmission Blocking routes of transmission may reduce the risk of hospital-acquired infection. Organisms may be transferred by the airborne route or by contact spread. Few organisms exist as isolated particles in air but many are carried on dust particles, which largely consist of skin scales. Staphylococci and other Gram-positive bacteria may be spread by air, particularly from patients or staff with infected lesions or those who shed increased numbers of epithelial cells. The airborne route may also spread respiratory viruses and bacteria during coughing or sneezing. Airborne spread may be controlled in two ways:

- the use of filtered air in ventilation systems, e.g. operating theatres
- isolation rooms or wards.

Patients with organisms that pose a risk for others are placed in **source isolation** to minimise spread. **Protective isolation** is provided for highly susceptible patients (e.g. immunosuppressed patients immediately following organ transplants). Ideally, isolation rooms should have pressurised ventilation systems which direct airflow in (for source isolation) or out of the room (for protective isolation).

Contact spread is transmission of organisms by direct contact between the patient and equipment or staff. This route is minimised by **aseptic technique**, taking particular care when handling dressings, secretions and excretions that may transmit organisms directly by hands or via contaminated equipment. However, any clinical contact with infected or colonised patients (or their immediate environment) may transfer organisms to the hands of staff. It is therefore very important that all staff are aware of the importance of **hand hygiene — the single most important aspect of infection control (Table 37.1 and Fig. 37.4)**.

III: Improve the patient's resistance to infection This may be achieved by:

- meticulous technique during surgery — haemostasis, removal of dead tissue and foreign bodies, avoiding wound drains where possible
- care of invasive devices, e.g. intravascular lines, urinary catheters and endotracheal tubes
- control of underlying disease, e.g. diabetes
- enhancing immunity by immunisation, e.g. tetanus
- avoiding unnecessary antimicrobial treatment
- appropriate use of antimicrobial prophylaxis.

TABLE 37.1

Hand hygiene

Social handwashing

Wet hands, wash with soap	Routine duties and before eating
Rinse and dry thoroughly	Visible contamination with excretions/secretions

Hygienic hand disinfection

Wash with antiseptic soap or detergent for 10–20 s	Before and after clinical contact with patients
or	
Alcohol hand rub (3 ml for 30 s)	

Surgical hand disinfection

Wash with antiseptic soap or detergent for 2 minutes	Before surgical procedures
or	
Alcohol hand rub (two applications of 5 ml amounts allowing first to dry)	

FIG 37.1 Main hospital-acquired infections

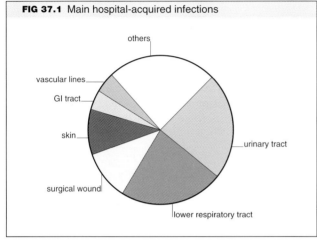

FIG 37.2 Specialities with higher prevalence rates of hospital-acquired infections

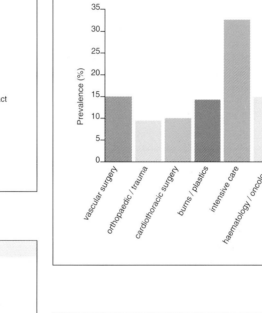

FIG 37.3 Sources of hospital-acquired infection

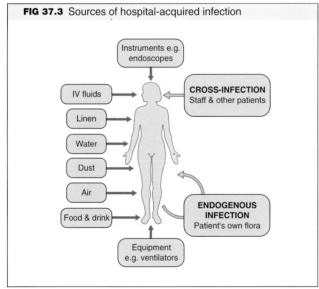

FIG 37.4 Areas commonly missed by inadequate handwashing

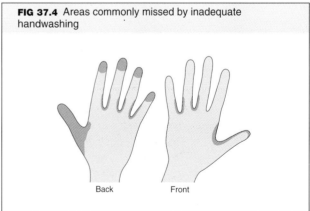

95

Case study 6

A previously fit 63 year old man is admitted for elective repair of an abdominal aortic aneurysm. Surgery is successful and he is transferred to ITU where his early postoperative recovery is good. However, he starts to show signs of sepsis — he is pyrexial, total white cell count has risen from 7.4 to $18.1 \times 10^6/mm^3$ in 24 h and he is still being ventilated 72 h postoperatively. He had two doses of co-amoxiclav as prophylaxis for surgery, but is not currently on antibiotics.

Questions

1. What are the three most likely sources of the infection?

2. Which bacteria most commonly cause problems at these sites?

3. What would you do now?

   There is an area of erythema surrounding his wound, but no evidence of a collection and only a slight serous discharge; a swab is taken for bacterial culture. There are a few fine crepitations on listening to his chest, and an X-ray is reported as 'suggesting left ventricular failure, although not excluding infection'; an aspirate from his endotracheal tube looks clean, but is sent for bacterial culture. He is catheterised, but his urine is completely clear; as it is negative for leucocyte esterase and nitrites on dipstick testing, a sample is not sent to the laboratory.

4. How would you treat this patient?

   His condition does not improve and, 48 h later, both blood cultures and the wound swab are reported as growing 'MRSA'.

5. How would you manage this man (RJ) now?

6. MRSA has not been isolated on any ITU patient previously — what would you do to assess the situation?

   A patient (AF) who was on the ward when RJ was admitted, was found to be MRSA screen positive; she had had multiple previous admissions to a number of hospitals with respiratory failure. Two other patients, admitted after RJ, were also found to be positive.

7. How would you manage this situation?

8. How might this outbreak have been avoided?

Answers

1. & 2. This is a surgical, hospital-acquired or 'nosocomial' infection.

Site of infection	Most common cause
• wound	*Staphylococcus aureus* β-haemolytic *Streptococcus* species
• respiratory tract	*Streptococcus pneumoniae* *Haemophilus influenzae* coliforms
• urinary tract	coliforms

3. You must assess, investigate appropriately and only then modify treatment if needed. As he is showing signs of systemic sepsis, two sets of peripheral blood cultures would be appropriate, together with cultures taken through any intravascular lines. Site-specific measures are described above.

4. The most probable source is his wound and therefore either flucloxacillin or cefuroxime would be reasonable cover against the most likely organisms. However, given that ventilator-associated pneumonia cannot be excluded, cefuroxime would be a better initial choice because of its broader spectrum of activity.

5. RJ is *systemically infected* and should be treated with a glycopeptide antibiotic such as vancomycin, to which MRSA is almost always sensitive. However, he may also be *colonised* at topical sites, so swabs should be taken from his nose, perineum, axillae and any broken areas of skin; if these grow MRSA, he will require a programme of disinfectant bathing. He should be placed in a side-room in 'standard isolation' to reduce the risk of spread to others.

6. Initially, the other patients on the ITU should be screened at the topical sites mentioned above to see if the source for this infection can be determined.

7. Each of the individual MRSA-positive patients would need to be managed in isolation as described for RJ. However, as this cluster is the first time that MRSA has been found on the unit, most teams would manage this quite aggressively to prevent MRSA becoming an endemic problem in a critical care unit. An outbreak committee might be formed and elective surgical admissions to the ITU stopped given the evidence of ongoing inter-patient transmission. The staff might be screened for MRSA carriers, and there would need to be a re-education campaign to improve the standards of hygienic procedures. The ward would need rigorous cleaning and it would be wise to introduce a policy of placing inter-hospital transfers into side-rooms whilst awaiting the results of an MRSA screen.

8. The three most important measures in effective infection control are hand-washing, hand-washing and hand-washing!

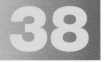

Sterilisation and disinfection

Sterilisation and disinfection are routinely used in hospitals and laboratories to eliminate or control the presence of potentially pathogenic micro-organisms for the protection of patients and staff. The two procedures are distinct and should not be confused:

- **Sterilisation** is the process by which all micro-organisms are removed or killed.
- **Disinfection** is the process by which vegetative, but not all, micro-organisms are removed or killed.

The choice of sterilisation or disinfection is dictated by the infection risk and may be defined as **high, intermediate** or **low (Table 38.1)**.

Physical cleaning with detergents (**sanitisers**) is often sufficient to remove microbes and organic material on which they thrive. It is also a prerequisite to effective sterilisation or disinfection.

Sterilisation

Sterilisation is used when the inactivation of all micro-organisms is an absolute requirement. This is achieved by **physical, chemical** or **mechanical** means (**Table 38.2**). Dry or moist heat are the most commonly used methods in hospitals and laboratories.

Dry heat Dry heat is only suitable for items able to withstand temperatures of at least 160°C and is used to sterilise glassware and metal instruments. Complete combustion in high-temperature incinerators is used for the disposal of human tissues and contaminated waste:

- hot air ovens at 160–180°C for 1 h
- incineration at >1000°C

Moist heat Moist heat sterilisation uses lower temperatures than dry heat and can better penetrate porous loads. The most effective and commonly used method is **autoclaving**. Autoclaves are similar to domestic pressure cookers, operating on the principle that water under pressure boils at a higher temperature. For example, at 15 psi the steam forms at 121°C and is sufficient to kill all micro-organisms, including spores.

Boiling at 100°C for 5 min will kill vegetative organisms, but spores can survive.

Pasteurisation at 63°C for 30 min or 72°C for 20 s is used in the food industry to eliminate vegetative pathogenic micro-organisms that can be transmitted in milk and other dairy products (e.g. *Mycobacteria, Salmonella, Campylobacter* and *Brucella*). It also prolongs the shelf-life of products by removing spoilage organisms (see also *ultra-heat treated* (UHT) milk, **Table 38.2**).

Chemical and physical For items that would be damaged by heat, other methods employing irradiation or chemical treatment are used. Examples include:

- gamma irradiation
- ultraviolet light
- glutaraldehyde liquid
- ethylene oxide gas
- formaldehyde gas.

Micro-organisms can also be physically removed from solutions by trapping them on porous membrane filters. However, viruses may pass through the pores.

Control of sterilisation In dry and moist heat sterilisation, it is critical that adequate temperature and exposure times are attained. This will vary with the nature and size of the load:

- Thermocouples with chart recorders give a visual record that the correct temperature and holding time were achieved during the sterilisation cycle.
- Browne's tubes and autoclave tape contain a chemical that changes colour when exposed to various temperatures.
- Paper strips impregnated with heat-resistant *Bacillus stearothermophilis* spores can be placed inside autoclave loads: spore survival indicates a problem with the autoclave process.

Disinfection

Disinfection is used to contain the presence of micro-organisms, usually for the purpose of infection control. Disinfectants have a limited spectrum of antimicrobial activity, notably the inability to kill bacterial spores, and cannot be used to guarantee sterility. The efficacy of many disinfectants is also limited by their corrosive and potentially toxic nature, and rapid inactivation by organic matter.

Disinfectants that can be applied directly to human skin to prevent, or possibly treat, infections are termed **antiseptics**. Others, termed **biocides**, are used in industrial applications to control microbial fouling and the presence of potentially pathogenic micro-organisms such as *Legionella pneumophila* in water-cooling towers.

Chlorine-and phenolic-based disinfectants are most widely used in hospitals and laboratories. **Appendix 7**, p. 131 lists some common disinfectants and antiseptics, their spectrum of microbial activity and application.

Examples of disinfectant use include:

- surface and floor cleaners
- containment of potentially infectious spillages
- skin and wound cleansing (antiseptics)
- treatment of drinking and bathing waters
- contact lens hygiene
- industrial processes (biocides).

TABLE 38.1

Categorisation of infection risk to patients and staff

Risk	Application	Requirement	Examples
High	Introduction into sterile body area	Sterilisation	Surgical instruments; single-use medical items (needles, syringes)
	Close contact with mucous membranes or damaged skin		Dressings, suturing thread
	Disposal of infectious waste		Laboratory cultures, human tissues and contaminated waste
Intermediate	Contact with mucous membranes	Disinfection (although sterilisation may be desirable)	Thermometers, respiratory apparatus, gastroscopes, endoscopes
	Contaminated with pathogenic microbes		Laboratory discard waste, patient bedpans, urinals
	Prior to use on immunocompromised patients		Protecting patient from microbes normally non-pathogenic to the immunocompetent person
Low	In contact with healthy skin	Sanitising (cleaning)	Patient trolleys, wheel chairs, beds
	No patient contact		Walls, floors, sinks, drains; in operating theatres disinfection may be used

TABLE 38.2

Examples of commonly used sterilisation methods

Method	Example	Mode of action	Application
Dry heat	Heating in a flame: hot air oven at 160–180°C for 1 h; incineration at >1000°C	Direct oxidisation	Inoculating loops; metal instruments and glassware; disposal of infectious waste
Moist heat	Autoclaving: 121°C for 15 min or 134°C for 3 min	Protein denaturation	Preparation of surgical instruments and dressings; production of laboratory culture media and reagents; disposal of infectious waste
	Boiling: 100°C for 5 min		Spores will survive; not suitable for sterilisation
	Steaming: 100°C for 5 min on 3 consecutive days (Tyndallisation)		Named after its originator: in a suitable liquid, spores will germinate on cooling and are then killed by the next day's steaming (the third heating is for extra security)
	Pasteurisation: 63°C for 30 min or 72°C for 20 s		Treatment of milk to remove pathogenic and food spoilage micro-organisms
	Ultra-heat treated (UHT) milk: 135–150°C		Treatment of milk to give indefinite shelf-life
Irradiation	Cobalt-60 gamma irradiation	Damage of DNA through free-radical formation	Heat-labile items such as plastic syringes, needles and other small single-use items
Chemical	Ethylene oxide gas	Alkylating agents causing protein and nucleic acid damage	Toxic and potentially explosive; used for items that cannot withstand autoclaving (e.g. heart valves)
	Formaldehyde gas		Toxic and irritant; decontamination of microbiology laboratory rooms and safety cabinets
	Glutaraldehyde		Toxic and irritant; decontamination of laboratory equipment and instruments (e.g. endoscopes)
Filtration	Passing solutions through a defined pore-sized membrane (e.g. 0.2 μm-0.45 μm)	Physical removal of microbes	Preparation of laboratory culture media, reagents and some pharmaceutical products

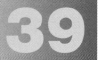

Food, water and public health microbiology

The environment is a major source of infection (**Fig. 39.1**). Surface soil has over 10^7 bacteria and 10^5 fungi in every gram, and even though most will not be harmful, many potential pathogens will be found. The advent of penicillin and other antibiotics, or even vaccination, have not been the factors most responsible for reducing the prevalence and incidence of infections. It has been the massive improvement in environmental hygiene.

Food microbiology Fresh foods are easily contaminated. Vegetables and fruit have soil contamination and, even after washing, they may harbour microbes that may have been in the washing water: outbreaks of hepatitis A and gastroenteritis have occurred with imported fruit that has been washed in 'river' water. Muscle is sterile, but meat is contaminated as it is prepared either through exposure to gut flora or because the machinery itself is contaminated. For example, the mechanical de-feathering of chickens adds *Salmonella* spp. to the chickens. Shellfish pose a particular hazard if grown in sewage-contaminated waters as they filter-feed and concentrate microbes.

Refrigeration at 5°C or lower retards bacterial growth, although those that are cold-adapted — **psychrophiles** and **psychrotrophs** (**Table 39.1**) — will eventually cause food spoilage. A number of other measures are also utilised to preserve food for longer in developed countries where food may take weeks from being harvested to reaching the table (**Table 39.2**).

Although not possible for all foods, the safest approach to preventing food poisoning is adequate cooking, as pathogens do not survive sustained high temperatures. Cooking may be compromised by poor handling so that the food is then re-contaminated. Control of food that is sold is regulated under the Food Safety Act 1990 (and other more specific legislation) in the UK; most food poisoning now results from poor handling after it is sold.

Water microbiology Risk to human health from water comes from either potable ('drinking') water or recreational waters. Both of these are controlled by legislation. Drinking water in most parts of developed countries is treated with chlorine-based compounds so that bacteria do not survive. Surveys have shown that less than 15% of potable water is used as cold drink, most consumption is with tea and other hot beverages. Illness does, however, occur when there is failure of the treatment process or when local water supplies, such as wells, are used.

Less stringent standards have to be used for recreational waters such as swimming baths, and natural bathing waters such as coastal resorts. Similarly most people are not at major risk of illness from water recreational activity, unless they spend much time with their heads immersed in natural waters or there is failure of treatment.

Air microbiology Respiratory-borne infections are common, and their increased incidence in winter months is thought to be partly attributable to people spending more time together indoors. This source of infection has been enhanced by the use of air conditioning which allows micro-organisms that flourish in the network to be spread within buildings. A prime example is *Legionella pneumophila*, which thrives in the warm water of ponds in cooling towers. In hospital theatres, air-borne transmission of microbes is controlled by filtering the entering air. Aerobiological monitoring is undertaken in circumstances of failure.

Public health microbiology This encompasses air, food, water and waste microbiology. The aims are to prevent and control infectious disease. Although there are dedicated health care professionals, such as consultants in communicable disease control and consultants in public health under the direction of the Director of Public Health, many doctors play a role. Prevention consists of several possible components (**Table 39.3**). Effective control of outbreaks of infection implies prompt diagnosis, descriptive epidemiology (including source(s) of infection, route of transmission, identification of people at risk) and rapid institution of effective measures to abort the outbreak. This should involve an outbreak control committee.

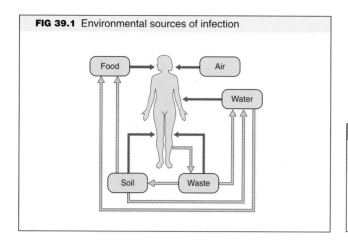

FIG 39.1 Environmental sources of infection

TABLE 39.1
Some common medically important psychrotrophs

- *Clostridium botulinum*
- *Yersinia* spp.
- *Listeria monocytogenes*
- *Aeromonas hydrophila*

TABLE 39.2	
Basic measures used in food preservation	
Method	**Example**
Complete removal of food-spoilage micro-organisms with maintenance of asepsis	Canning involves temperatures of 115°C for 25–100 min intervals; not absolutely effective
Low temperature	Refrigeration, freezing 'Cook-chill'
High temperature	Pasteurisation
Water removal	Lyophilisation
Decreased water availability	Addition of sugar, salt or other solutes
Chemicals	Addition of nitrates, organic acids
Irradiation	Use of UV or gamma-irradiation

TABLE 39.3
General measures for the prevention of infectious disease

- Education
- Adequate nutrition
- Hygienic living conditions
- High level of water sanitation
- Effective waste disposal
- Immunisation
- Prompt control of outbreaks of infection

40 Antibacterials — the principles

Antimicrobial chemotherapy exploits the differences between micro-organisms and host cells. Agents that attack specific targets unique to micro-organisms are thus relatively safe to the host — the concept of 'selective toxicity'. Strictly speaking the term 'antibiotic' refers to naturally occurring products which inhibit or kill micro-organisms. It is, however, often used to describe chemically modified or synthetic agents that are more correctly called 'antibacterial' or 'antimicrobial' agents.

Antibacterials may be classified by their target site of action (**Fig. 40.1** and **Table 40.1**). **Bacteriostatic** antibacterials inhibit bacterial growth, whereas those that kill bacteria are termed **bactericidal**. For many agents, bactericidal activity is species-dependent and generally not essential except in some immune-suppressed individuals and in cases of endocarditis.

Some agents are **narrow-spectrum** and mainly active against a limited range of bacteria (e.g. penicillin activity against Gram-positive bacteria or gentamicin activity against Gram-negatives). **Broad-spectrum** agents such as cefuroxime and ciprofloxacin are active against a wide range of bacteria. Such agents are clinically useful, but extensive usage is likely to encourage resistance by inducing or selecting resistant strains.

Antibacterial resistance

Some bacteria show inherent or **innate resistance** to certain antibiotics (e.g. *Pseudomonas aeruginosa* is always resistant to benzylpenicillin). Other bacteria have **acquired resistance** as a result of genetic change (e.g. some strains of *Streptococcus pneumoniae* are now resistant to penicillin). Significant increases in bacterial resistance have been seen recently, and some strains of staphylococci, streptococci and Gram-negative rods have been identified that are resistant to all currently available antibacterials.

Resistance may result from **chromosomal mutation** or **transmissible ('infectious') drug resistance** (**Fig. 40.2**). Spontaneous mutation of the chromosome may change protein synthesis to create bacteria that have a selective advantage and will therefore outgrow the susceptible population.

Plasmids are extra-chromosomal loops of DNA, which replicate independently but can be incorporated back into the chromosome. Those plasmids that code for antimicrobial resistance are called **resistance (or R) factors**. A single plasmid may confer resistance to many antibacterials and can move between species (**Fig. 40.3**). Gram-negative plasmids are generally spread by **conjugation**, where genes pass between bacterial cells joined by sex pili. Such plasmids often confer resistance to many different antimicrobials. Gram-positive plasmids are usually spread by

transduction — genetic transfer via viruses that infect bacteria (bacteriophages) — and the resulting resistance is generally confined to one or two agents only.

Transposons ('jumping genes') are non-replicating pieces of DNA, which jump between one plasmid and another and between plasmids and the chromosome.

Mechanisms of resistance

There are three main resistance mechanisms. **Alteration in the target site** reduces or eliminates the binding of the drug (e.g. erythromycin resistance in staphylococci and streptococci). With **altered permeability**, transport of the antimicrobial into the cell is reduced (e.g. in some types of aminoglycoside resistance) or the drug is actively pumped out of the cell e.g. tetracycline resistance. Finally the antimicrobial may be modified or destroyed by **inactivating enzymes** (e.g. β-lactamases which attack penicillins and cephalosporins).

Pharmacology

Some antibiotics have excellent **absorption** by the oral route (e.g. ampicillin), others are only partially absorbed (e.g. penicillin V) and others not absorbed at all (e.g. gentamicin). In some cases non-absorbable agents are used to act against enteric organisms (e.g. vancomycin and *Clostridium difficile*). Metronidazole achieves good serum and tissue levels by the rectal route. In acute serious infections the **parenteral** (intravenous or intramuscular) route is generally used to administer antibacterials.

The antibacterial must achieve sufficient **distribution** to reach the site of infection. Factors such as lipid solubility, protein-binding, intracellular penetration and the ability to cross the blood–CSF and blood–brain barriers affect distribution.

The **half-life** will influence the dosage interval, and **metabolism** and **excretion** may affect the choice of agent especially in patients with impaired renal or hepatic function.

Toxicity

Despite the principle of 'selective toxicity', adverse reactions occur in about 5% of antibacterial courses. Commoner reactions include self-limiting gastrointestinal upset (especially diarrhoea) and mild but irritating skin rashes. However, severe and potentially life-threatening complications are well documented and include: anaphylaxis, impairment of hepatic or renal function, neuro- and oto-toxicity, bone marrow suppression, pseudomembranous colitis and Stevens–Johnson syndrome.

TABLE 40.1

Classes of antibacterials

Target site	Antibacterial class	Example agents	Comments/adverse reactions
Cell wall	β-Lactams		
	Penicillins	Benzylpenicillin, ampicillin	Generally safe but allergic reactions
	Cephalosporins	Cephalexin, cefuroxime, ceftazidime	Broad-spectrum: overusage promotes resistance
	Glycopeptides	Vancomycin, teicoplanin	Vancomycin may be nephro/oto-toxic, assay required
	Carbapenems	Imipenem, meropenem	Reserved for resistant pathogens
Protein synthesis	Aminoglycosides	Gentamicin, amikacin	Potential nephro- and oto-toxicity; assay required
	Tetracyclines	Tetracycline, doxycycline	Stain teeth and bone
	Chloramphenicol	Chloramphenicol	Potential marrow toxicity
	Macrolides	Erythromycin	Often used in penicillin-allergic patients
	Lincosamides	Clindamycin	Associated with pseudomembranous colitis
	Fusidic acid	Fusidic acid	May cause jaundice
Nucleic acid synthesis	Sulphonamides	Sulphamethoxazole	Rarely used because of toxic reactions
	Trimethoprim	Trimethoprim	Mainly used in treatment of UTI
	Quinolones	Nalidixic acid, ciprofloxacin	Early quinolones have limited Gram-positive activity
	Rifamycins	Rifampicin	Stains tears/urine, may cause jaundice
	Nitroimidazoles	Metronidazole	Antabuse effect with alcohol
Cell membrane function	Polymyxins	Colistin	Used for bowel decontamination or by inhalation
Others unknown		Nitrofurantoin	Urinary activity only
		Isoniazid	Antituberculous agents
		Ethambutol	

FIG 40.1 Antibacterial sites of action

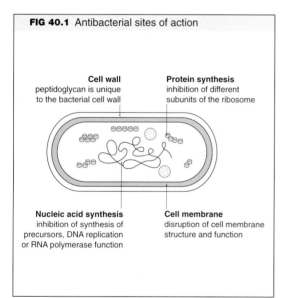

Cell wall
peptidoglycan is unique to the bacterial cell wall

Protein synthesis
inhibition of different subunits of the ribosome

Nucleic acid synthesis
inhibition of synthesis of precursors, DNA replication or RNA polymerase function

Cell membrane
disruption of cell membrane structure and function

FIG 40.2 Mutational and transmissible resistance

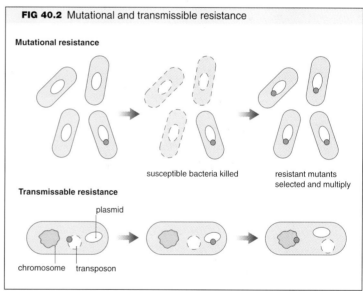

Mutational resistance

susceptible bacteria killed

resistant mutants selected and multiply

Transmissable resistance

plasmid

chromosome   transposon

FIG 40.3 Transduction and conjugation

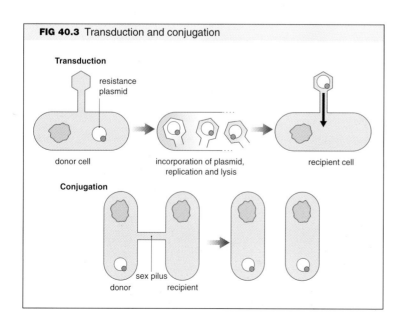

Transduction

resistance plasmid

donor cell

incorporation of plasmid, replication and lysis

recipient cell

Conjugation

sex pilus

donor   recipient

Antibacterial therapy — the practice

41

The aim of successful antibacterial therapy is to select the right agent, dose, route and duration using laboratory data where and when available. The reality is that up to 30% of antibacterial prescriptions may be unnecessary because:

- there is no clear evidence of infection
- the infection does not require antibacterials, e.g. viral respiratory tract infections
- the wrong agent has been chosen.

There are now over 80 antibacterials available on the British market, and making a rational selection for a particular patient requires a logical approach. In practice many prescriptions are based simply on the suspected site of infection, e.g. respiratory or urinary tract. A more appropriate selection is based on a combination of clinical and laboratory findings, refining the choice by considering specific patient and drug factors as shown in **Fig. 41.1**. Whenever possible, appropriate specimens should be collected before antibacterial therapy is started.

Rational antibacterial usage can be categorised as

- initial **empirical** therapy ('best guess' or 'blind')
- specific or **definitive** treatment (generally directed by laboratory reports)
- **prophylaxis** (see below).

In the following situations it may be appropriate to consider combined therapy:

- broad-spectrum cover when
  (a) the pathogen is unknown, e.g. septicaemia
  (b) multiple pathogens are possible, e.g. perforated large bowel
- to prevent emergence of resistance, e.g. anti-tuberculous therapy
- to provide enhanced activity, e.g. treatment of infective endocarditis with penicillin and gentamicin. Such a combination is said to be **synergistic** — the activity is greater than the sum of the individual activities. When two antibacterials significantly interfere with each other the combination is **antagonistic**.

It is important to minimise unnecessary prescriptions, because all antibacterial usage may be associated with

- unwanted effects, e.g. rash, diarrhoea
- increasing costs — antibacterials typically account for around 15% of the drug costs of a teaching hospital.
- increasing resistance in both Gram-positive and Gram-negative species.

Antibacterials are unique in that they have an impact on the population as well as the individual patient for whom they were prescribed. Increasing (and frequently unnecessary) use of antibacterials is leading to a corresponding increase in bacterial resistance. Following the significant increase in resistance rates in Gram-negative bacteria, we have now seen a recent increase in multiply resistant Gram-positive bacteria — notably methicillin-resistant *Staph. aureus* (MRSA) and vancomycin-resistant enterococci (VRE). This has lead to the fear of a post-antibiotic era where many infections may be untreatable.

The recommended **duration** of antibacterial therapy has decreased over recent years. For many acute infections, treatment for 5–7 days is often adequate, and many uncomplicated urinary tract infections will respond to 3 day regimens. In endocarditis and infections of bone and joints, therapy is continued for several weeks, and successful treatment of tuberculosis requires at least 6 months of combination therapy.

Laboratory aspects

Susceptibility testing is readily available for most antibacterial agents and generally distinguishes isolates as **sensitive** or **resistant** (although the term **intermediate** is sometimes used) (**Fig. 41.2**). In some circumstances (e.g. infective endocarditis) a quantitative result is required and this is usually reported as a minimum inhibitory concentration (**MIC**). Such reports are helpful when comparing the susceptibility of the isolate with antibiotic concentrations achievable in the blood or at the specific site of infection.

Some antibacterials such as gentamicin and vancomycin have a narrow **therapeutic index** — the margin between therapeutic and potentially toxic concentrations is small. To ensure that safe and effective concentrations are achieved with these agents, **antibacterial assays** are performed (**Fig. 41.3**).

Prophylaxis is defined as the use of antimicrobial agents to prevent infection in susceptible patients. The majority of antibacterial prophylaxis is employed in surgery, although there are a few medical indications (**Table 41.1**). The principles of surgical prophylaxis are:

- It must be an adjunct to good surgical technique.
- The infection to be prevented occurs
  (a) frequently (e.g. large bowel surgery)
  (b) rarely but with disastrous consequences, e.g. cardiac valve surgery.
- Likely pathogens and susceptibilities are predictable.
- Agents have proven efficacy.
- Route and timing ensure adequate concentrations at time of practice.
- Duration of prophylaxis is generally < 24 h — usually a single dose.

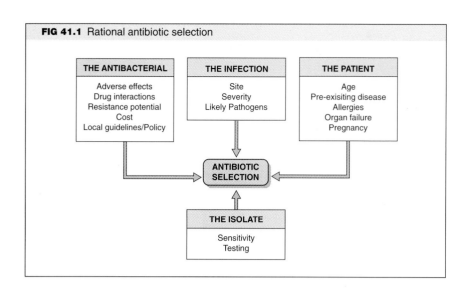

FIG 41.1 Rational antibiotic selection

THE ANTIBACTERIAL	THE INFECTION	THE PATIENT
Adverse effects	Site	Age
Drug interactions	Severity	Pre-exisiting disease
Resistance potential	Likely Pathogens	Allergies
Cost		Organ failure
Local guidelines/Policy		Pregnancy

ANTIBIOTIC SELECTION

THE ISOLATE

Sensitivity Testing

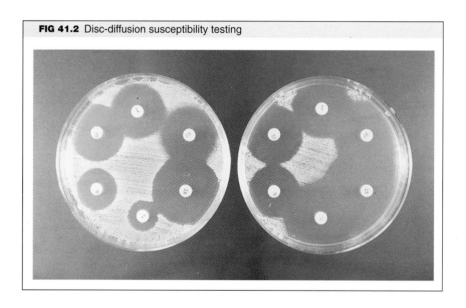

FIG 41.2 Disc-diffusion susceptibility testing

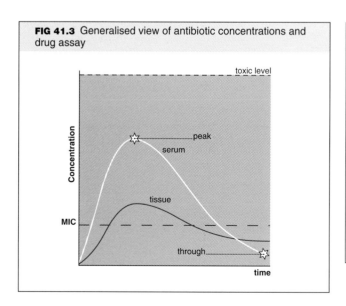

FIG 41.3 Generalised view of antibiotic concentrations and drug assay

toxic level

peak

serum

tissue

MIC

through

Concentration

time

TABLE 41.1

Examples of antibacterial prophylaxis

Category	Indication
Medical	Prevent recurrent streptococcal disease following rheumatic fever
	Eradicate carriage of *N. meningitidis* in close contacts of cases of meningococcal disease
	Prevent tuberculosis in asymptomatic contacts
Surgical	Prevent infective endocarditis in patients with damaged valves undergoing dental or other surgery
	Abdominal surgery
	Vascular surgery
	Orthopaedic implant surgery
	Gynaecological surgery
	Lower-limb amputation
	Cardiac surgery

Case study 7

A previously fit 66 year old widower presents to his GP with a fever and non-productive cough. He has recently returned from a trip to Spain to visit his son. Examination confirms a raised temperature and pulse rate but no signs in the chest. The GP prescribes oral amoxicillin.

The patient phones the next day, as he is feeling worse, and the GP visits. He finds the patient systemically stable but with a continuing fever. The GP changes the antibiotic to cephalexin.

Questions

1. Can a reliable diagnosis be made from the clinical findings given?

2. If this is a lower respiratory tract infection, was the initial antibiotic choice reasonable?

3. What explanations might be given for the failure to respond?

4. Was the antibiotic change appropriate?

   A neighbour phones the GP later that day. The patient now seems very unwell, and the GP revisits and immediately arranges hospital admission. Chest X-ray shows right middle lobe infiltration. A diagnosis of pneumonia is made, and blood cultures and sputum culture are arranged. Treatment is changed to i.v. cefuroxime and clarithromycin.

   A blood gas determination that evening prompts admission to the ITU. Sputum culture the next day shows *Strep. pneumoniae*.

5. The microbiologist recommends a change of antibiotics — why?

   Sensitivity testing of the isolate confirms significantly-reduced susceptibility to penicillin. However, despite appropriate therapy with ceftriaxone and intensive support including ventilation, the patient's condition deteriorates. Chest X-ray now shows extensive shadowing, and tracheal secretions are profuse. Culture shows *Pseudomonas aeruginosa*.

6. How should the antibiotic therapy be modified?

   Treatment is changed to ceftazidime. The patient's condition stabilises, but 3 days later fever returns and respiratory function worsens. Cultures of central line blood, peripheral blood and tracheal aspirate are taken.

7. What empirical changes to antibiotic therapy should be considered?

   Blood cultures taken through the central line grow *Enterococcus faecium*. The tracheal aspirate now yields a *Ps. aeruginosa* isolate resistant to ceftazidime. Vancomycin is started, but the patient dies of multi-organ failure the next day.

8. Are all strains of enterococci susceptible to vancomycin?

9. Is the emergence of resistance to ceftazidime unusual?

Answers

1. Cough suggests a respiratory tract infection, but the findings are non-specific. Typhoid is unusual in Spain but might present this way in travellers from endemic areas. If this is a respiratory tract infection, the site cannot be ascertained (bronchitis, pneumonia).

2. In a patient without obstructive airways disease, acute viral bronchitis or bacterial pneumonia should be considered. Amoxicillin is a reasonable first choice agent for the latter. (Travel to Spain is a clue to specific problems with antibiotic resistance that are probably not appreciated by most GPs — see 5 below.)

3. Possibilities include:

   — wrong diagnosis
   — wrong antibiotic (antibiotic resistance)
   — wrong dose
   — wrong route
   — patient did not take the antibiotic (compliance)
   — too early to judge response.

4. First-generation cephalosporins are inappropriate antibiotics for respiratory tract infections, as they are not effective against *Haemophilus* spp. One day is too soon to judge response, but if a change were to be made, use of a macrolide to cover atypical infections (especially *Legionella*, given the travel history) should be considered.

5. Penicillin-insensitive strains are common in Spain and ceftriaxone/cefotaxime would be a wise choice.

6. This may represent colonisation following broad-spectrum antibiotics that inhibit the normal respiratory flora and allow overgrowth of Gram-negatives. If there are new chest X-ray changes, *Pseudomonas* should be considered a pathogen in a ventilated patient, and an antipseudomonal agent should be started — for example:

   — antipseudomonal β-lactam (e.g. piperacillin, ceftazidime, or meropenem, all +/− gentamicin)
   — or quinolone (e.g. ciprofloxacin) +/− gentamicin.

7. Emergence of resistance of *Pseudomonas* or a new infection, e.g. line-associated infection, should be considered. Changing ceftazidime to ciprofloxacin or meropenem would be reasonable. Vancomycin might be used to cover Gram-positive line-associated infection, but a line change should be considered.

8. Vancomycin-resistant enterococci (VRE) are now well recognised. The use of ceftazidime would select for enterococci that are inherently resistant to cephalosporins.

9. Third-generation cephalosporins are renowned for their potential to induce or select resistant Gram-negative bacteria, especially pseudomonads.

42 Antiviral therapy

The replication of viruses depends on the use of the biochemical machinery of the host cell. Selectivity of antiviral drugs is, therefore, harder to achieve than with antibacterial drugs. There are, however, several aspects of the virus replication cycle that can be targeted (**Fig. 42.1**). Optimal therapy depends on rapid diagnosis, and this is particularly difficult when the virus has a long incubation period or prodrome. Latent viruses also prove relatively resistant to antiviral therapy.

Treatment of herpesviruses

Aciclovir (acycloguanosine) and its derivatives are the mainstay of treatment of herpes simplex virus infections. Aciclovir is a nucleoside analogue that requires conversion to a triphosphate to be active. The first phosphate group is added by herpesvirus-coded thymidine kinase which ensures selectivity for virally infected cells. Two further phosphates are added by cellular kinases to produce an inhibitor of DNA polymerase. It is also a substrate of the enzyme and incorporated in place of guanosine triphosphate but, because it lacks an essential hydroxyl group, causes termination of elongation of the DNA chain. Two newer derivatives of aciclovir, **penciclovir** and **valaciclovir**, have additional clinical activity against varicella-zoster virus. Ganciclovir is clinically active against cytomegalovirus.

Treatment of HIV-1

Nucleoside analogues have also been developed for the treatment of asymptomatic and symptomatic AIDS, and post-exposure prophylaxis (**Table 42.1**). These act as inhibitors of viral reverse transcriptase (RT). Specificity is poor, so that all these drugs are toxic: bone marrow suppression, pancreatitis and myositis are not uncommon and may be dose-related. Rapid evolution of the virus has also meant that resistance inevitably develops. As resistance to a specific drug is coded for by particular genetic mutations, this has been minimised by the use of combination of nucleoside analogues. Optimal combination therapy also uses other classes of drugs which interfere with different parts of the replication cycle.

Non-nucleoside RT inhibitors and drugs that inhibit the action of the viral protease have also been developed for use in combination with nucleoside analogues (**Table 42.1**). They are not without serious side effects, and resistance also develops to these drugs.

This area of drug development is particularly rapid, and new classes of drugs are anticipated.

Other antiviral agents

Ribavirin is a nucleoside analogue that has broad-spectrum in-vitro activity. Its main use has been for severe RSV infections in children, particularly those with congenital cardiopulmonary disorders. It is also useful clinically in patients with severe influenza B and Lassa fever.

Amantadine and **rimantadine** inhibit the uncoating and egress of influenza A. They have no effect against influenza B or C, and their use, particularly in the elderly, is associated with minor neurological side effects (headache, confusion, etc.). New, less toxic drugs that inhibit the viral neuraminidase, an enzyme essential for virus entry into a cell, offer therapy with less-toxic side effects.

Interferons (**Fig 42.2**) when discovered were hoped to be the 'magic bullet' for viruses. They are agents produced naturally in response to viral infection. High local doses are, however, difficult to deliver therapeutically, and use is currently limited to the management of chronic hepatitis B and C and papillomavirus infections. Viral eradication does not occur in these conditions, and infection tends to recur when therapy is stopped. The use of newer agents, such as famciclovir and lamivudine, in the treatment of chronic hepatitis B shows promise and may form the basis of better combination therapy of this condition.

Phosphonoformate is an anti-herpes drug which is used as an alternative to aciclovir if resistance to the latter develops or to ganciclovir in cytomegalovirus treatment. It has an unusual side effect of causing penile ulcers.

There have been many drugs, such as pirodavir for rhinovirus and antisense therapy for human papillomavirus infections, which have an in-vitro but not in-vivo effect. Drug engineering is likely, however, to produce chemical derivatives which enhance the latter.

Monitoring of antiviral therapy

Antiviral resistance has emerged with the more widespread use of antivirals. Antiviral susceptibility testing methods are now available if clinical resistance occurs, and, in future, antiviral load measurements will be developed. Clinical resistance does not, however, equate with lack of in-vitro susceptibility of an isolate to the drug.

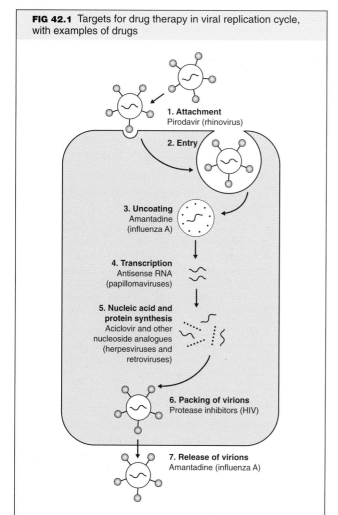

FIG 42.1 Targets for drug therapy in viral replication cycle, with examples of drugs

1. Attachment
Pirodavir (rhinovirus)

2. Entry

3. Uncoating
Amantadine
(influenza A)

4. Transcription
Antisense RNA
(papillomaviruses)

**5. Nucleic acid and
protein synthesis**
Aciclovir and other
nucleoside analogues
(herpesviruses and
retroviruses)

6. Packing of virions
Protease inhibitors (HIV)

7. Release of virions
Amantadine (influenza A)

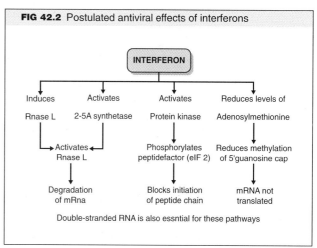

FIG 42.2 Postulated antiviral effects of interferons

INTERFERON

| Induces | Activates | Activates | Reduces levels of |

Rnase L | 2-5A synthetase | Protein kinase | Adenosylmethionine

Activates ← Rnase L

Phosphorylates
peptidefactor (eIF 2)

Reduces methylation
of 5'guanosine cap

Degradation
of mRna

Blocks initiation
of peptide chain

mRNA not
translated

Double-stranded RNA is also essntial for these pathways

TABLE 42.1

Drugs used in the treatment of HIV-1 infection

Nucleoside analogues	Azidothymidine (AZT)
	Dideoxycytidine (dDC)
	Dideoxyinosine (dDI)
	Stavudine (d4T)
	'Epivir' (3TC)
Non-nucleoside RT	Nevirapine
	Loviride
	Delarvidine
Protease inhibitors	Ritonavir
	Saquinavir
	Indinavir
	Nelfinavir

43

Antifungal therapy

Fungi are eukaryotic organisms and share many common biological and metabolic features with human cells. As a consequence, antifungal agents are potentially toxic to our own cells in their mode of action. This limits the number of compounds available for the treatment of human mycoses. In addition, many fungi also have detoxification mechanisms that remove the drugs.

Fungal infections are termed **mycoses** and these may be either **superficial** (localised to the epidermis, hair and nails), **subcutaneous** (confined to the dermis and subcutaneous tissue) or **systemic** (deep infections of the internal organs).

Superficial mycoses caused by dermatophytes are usually treated by application of creams or ointments to the infected area (**topical therapy**). Subcutaneous and systemic mycoses require oral or intravenous administration (**systemic therapy**). In vaginal candidiasis ('thrush'), treatment may be given using antifungal pessaries. Some antifungal agents are too toxic for systemic use but can be used safely in topical therapy of superficial mycoses. Antifungal agents are also used prophylactically in patients receiving immunosuppressive therapy to prevent infection by opportunistic fungi from the environment and the normal flora of the body. Examples are given below, and their uses are summarised in **Table 43.1**.

As with antibacterial drugs, many antifungal agents are derived from the fermentation products of certain fungi (e.g. *Streptomyces* and *Penicillium*). The principal targets and mode of action of antifungal drugs are through the disruption or inhibition of fungal:

- cell wall integrity
- cell wall biosynthesis
- RNA synthesis
- cell division and nucleic acid biosynthesis.

Polyenes These bind to sterol components (notably **ergosterol**) of the fungal cell membrane, causing increased permeability, leakage of cellular components and cell death:

- **Nystatin** is not absorbed by the gut and is too toxic for parenteral use. It is used as a topical preparation in the treatment of ophthalmic, oral and vaginal candidiasis.
- **Amphotericin B** is the most important member of the polyene antifungals. It is active against a wide range of fungi but not dermatophytes. It is the drug of choice in the treatment of systemic fungal infections. However, amphotericin B is potentially toxic and can result in renal damage. It is now commonly given as a liposomal preparation in which the drug is encapsulated in phospholipid-containing liposomes, thereby reducing toxicity.

Azoles These are synthetic compounds that inhibit ergosterol biosynthesis. They are an important class of antifungal agents, being effective in both superficial and systemic fungal infections, whilst showing reduced toxicity compared with amphotericin B:

- **fluconazole** — effective in the treatment of systemic candidiasis and cryptococcosis
- **itraconazole** — superficial, subcutaneous and systemic infections, including aspergillosis.

The following azoles are also sometimes used but have largely been superseded by the introduction of fluconazole and itraconazole:

- **ketoconazole** — topical therapy for dermatophyte and cutaneous candidiasis
- **miconazole** — topical therapy for dermatophyte and cutaneous candidiasis.

The following azole antifungals are also used in the topical treatment of superficial mycoses:

- **clotrimazole** — dermatophyte, oral, cutaneous and vaginal candidiasis
- **econazole nitrate** — dermatophyte, cutaneous and vaginal candidiasis
- **isoconazole** — vaginal candidiasis
- **sulconazole nitrate** — fungal skin infections.

Pyrimidines Synthetic analogues of pyrimidine, they are converted inside fungi to compounds that replace uracil in RNA synthesis and interfere with protein production:

- **Flucytosine (5-fluorocytosine)** is converted to 5-fluorouracil which becomes incorporated into the RNA, causing abnormalities in protein synthesis. Mainly used in the treatment of yeast infections. Drug resistance can arise during treatment. Usually used in combination with amphotericin B for the treatment of cryptococcosis, disseminated candidiasis and fungal endocarditis.

Benzofurans These act principally through the inhibition of cellular microtubule formation preventing mitosis (cell division). They also inhibit nucleic acid biosynthesis:

- **Griseofulvin** is the only medically useful agent of the group. Given orally, the drug is concentrated from the blood-stream into the stratum corneum of the skin. Hence it is used in the treatment of dermatophyte infections.

Allyamines These are new synthetic agents that act on fungal ergosterol synthesis:

- **Terbinafine** can be administered orally or topically in the treatment of dermatophyte and superficial candidiasis.

Cotrimoxazole Cotrimoxazole (trimethoprim plus sulphamethoxazole) is used in the treatment and prophylaxis of pneumocystis pneumonia.

TABLE 43.1

Summary of antifungal therapy

Infection	Antifungal agent	Route of administration	Comment
Superficial mycoses			
Dermatophytes (ringworm); pityriasis versicolor	Griseofulvin	Oral	Low toxicity but should not be used in patients with liver disease
	Terbinafine	Oral or topical	Low toxicity and highly effective
	Itraconazole	Oral	Minor side effects: headache, nausea, vomiting
Candidiasis	Fluconazole	Oral	Some *Candida* species, other than *C. albicans*, show innate resistance
	Nystatin	Topical	
	Clotrimazole	Topical	
	Itraconazole	Oral	
Subcutaneous mycoses			
Sporotrichosis	Amphotericin B	Oral, i.v. infusion	High risk of toxic reactions: fever, rigors, headache, vomiting, nephrotoxicity (long-term); reduced toxicity with liposomal preparations
	Terbinafine	Oral or topical	
	Itraconazole	Oral	
Systemic mycoses			
Candidiasis and cryptococcosis	Amphotericin B	Oral, i.v. infusion	
	Flucytosine + amphotericin B	Oral, i.v. infusion	Flucytosine is not used alone, as drug resistance can arise during treatment; may cause nausea, vomiting, neutropenia and jaundice
	Fluconazole	i.v. infusion	
Aspergillosis	Amphotericin B	Oral, i.v. infusion	
Histoplasmosis; blastomycosis; coccidioidomycosis; paracoccidioidomycosis	Ketoconazole (amphotericin B for coccidioidomycosis CNS involvement)	Oral	
Pneumocystis	Cotrimoxazole (trimethoprim + sulphamethoxazole)	Oral	Effective only against *Pneumocystis carinii*
	Pentamidine	i.m. and aerosolised	Toxic reactions when given i.m.

i.v., intravenous; i.m., intramuscular

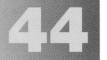

Antiprotozoal and antihelminthic therapy

Recent years have seen many advances in parasitology; however, the treatment of many infections remains unsatisfactory. Effective therapeutic agents are limited and of disappointing activity because:

- Similarities between parasite and human cells can result in drug side effects.
- Drugs may not be active against all biological forms of an organism (cyst and eggs are particularly resistant).
- Drug resistance has limited the effectiveness of many agents, particularly in malaria.
- There are no vaccines available against human parasites.

Antiprotozoal agents (Table 44.1)

Metronidazole is one of the nitro-imidazole antibiotics active only against anaerobic organisms. It is highly effective in the treatment of amoebiasis due to **Entamoeba histolytica**, trichomoniasis and giardiasis. It is also used to treat anaerobic bacterial infections. Inside the organism it is reduced to the active form, producing DNA damage. The related compound **tinidazole** is also effective against these protozoa.

Metronidazole is less effective against the cyst form of *E. histolytica*, and alternative agents such as **diloxanide furoate** are used to treat asymptomatic cyst excretors.

Melarsoprol is a trivalent arsenical active against African trypanosomiasis ('sleeping sickness'). It is thought to inhibit parasite pyruvate kinase and possibly other enzymes involved in glycolysis. Melarsoprol crosses the blood–brain barrier and is therefore effective in late stage disease when the trypanosomes have infected the central nervous system.

Pentamidine is a diamidine compound used in the early stages of African trypanosomiasis, some forms of leishmaniasis and pneumocystis pneumonia. It is thought to act by interacting with parasite DNA (particularly kinetoplast DNA of *Trypanosoma* and *Leishmania*), preventing cell division.

Nifurtimox is a nitrofuran active against American trypanosomiasis (Chagas' disease) in the acute phase of infection. It acts by forming toxic oxygen radicals within the parasite. The nitroimidazole derivative **benznidazole** is used as an alternative treatment.

Pentavalent antimony compounds (**stibogluconate** and **meglumine antimonate**) are used to treat leishmaniasis. However, sensitivity varies among species and geographic location. Their mode of action is uncertain but is thought to affect parasite metabolism.

Amphotericin B is an antifungal agent active against *Leishmania* and is used as an alternative to the antimonial compounds in the treatment of leishmaniasis. It is thought to alter parasite surface membrane permeability, causing leakage of intracellular components.

Antimalarial agents are discussed elsewhere (see Chapter 33).

Antihelminthic agents (Table 44.2)

Protozoa and helminths are physically and biologically distinct. Drugs active against one are not usually active against the other.

Albendazole is an antibiotic chemically related to metronidazole that has antihelminthic activity by conversion in the liver to the active form of albendazole sulphoxide. It is used to treat hookworms, strongyloidiasis, ascariasis, enterobiasis and trichuriasis. It has also proved effective in some microsporidial infections.

Mebendazole is a synthetic benzimidazole that is highly effective against hookworms, ascariasis, enterobiasis and trichuriasis. It acts by selectively binding to helminthic tubulin, preventing microtubule assembly. This results in parasite immobilisation and death. The related compound, **thiabendazole** is used in strongyloidiasis.

Diethylcarbamazine (DEC) is active against the microfilaria: bancroftian filariasis ('elephantiasis'), loaiasis ('eyeworm') and onchocerciasis ('river blindness'). DEC causes paralysis of the worms and also alters the surface membranes, resulting in enhanced killing by the host's immune system. However, therapy usually causes severe itching (Mazzotti reaction), and DEC is now considered too toxic for use.

Ivermectin has replaced DEC in the treatment of the microfilariae because of reduced toxicity. It is a macrolytic lactone which blocks the parasite neurotransmitter GABA, preventing nerve signalling and resulting in paralysis. The introduction of ivermectin has been a major advance in the treatment of onchocerciasis. It has also been shown to have good activity against nematodes and is increasingly being used in the treatment of strongyloidiasis.

Praziquantel is an isoquinoline derivative active against trematodes (flukes) and cestodes (tapeworms). In causes increased cell permeability to calcium ions, resulting in contraction and paralysis. In schistosomiasis, the trematodes are then swept to the liver where they are attacked by phagocytes. With cestodes, the tapeworm detaches from the gut wall and is expelled with the faeces.

Niclosamide is also used in the treatment of adult tapeworms although praziquantel is preferred as it is active against both larvae and adults of *Taenia solium* (pork tapeworm) and may prevent cysticercosis autoinfection.

TABLE 44.1

Common antiprotozoal drugs

Organism	Disease	Agent
Amoebae		
Entamoeba histolytica	Amoebiasis	Metronidazole, tinidazole, diloxanide furoate (asymptomatic cyst excretors)
Naegleria fowleri	Primary amoebic meningo-encephalitis (PAM)	Amphotericin B
Acanthamoeba	Encephalitis	Effective agent awaited
	Keratitis	Polyhexamethylene biguanide (PHMB) + propamidine isethionate
Flagellates		
Giardia lamblia	giardiasis	Metronidazole, tinidazole
Trichomonas vaginalis	trichomoniasis	Metronidazole, tinidazole
Ttrypanosmoma	African trypanosomiasis (sleeping sickness)	Pentamidine isethionate (early stages), melarsoprol (late stages when CNS involved)
	American trypanosomiasis (Chagas' disease)	Nifurtimox, benznidazole
Leishmania	Leishmaniasis	Stibogluconate, meglumine antimonate; amphotericin B, pentamidine isethionate (alternatives)
Apicomplexa		
Toxoplasma gondii	Toxoplasmosis	Pyrimethamine + sulphadiazine, spiramycin (in pregnancy and neonatal infection), azithromycin, atovaquone (cysticidal)
Cryptosporidium parvum	Cryptosporidiosis	Effective agent awaited

TABLE 44.2

Common antihelminthic drugs

Organism	Disease	Agent
Nematodes (worms)		
Necata americanis	Hookworm	Mebendazole, albendazole
Ancylostoma duodenale		
Strongyloides stericoralis	Strongyloidiasis	Thiabendazole, ivermectin
Ascaris lumbricoides	Ascariasis ('roundworm')	Mebendazole, albendazole
Toxocara canis and *T. cati*	Toxocariasis: visceral or ocular larval migrans	Diethylcarbamazine (DEC), mebendazole, albendazole
Trichuris trichiura	Trichurias ('whipworm')	Albendazole, mebendazole
Enterobius vermicularis	Enterobiasis ('pinworm'/'threadworm')	Albendazole, mebendazole
Filaria		
Wuchereria bancrofti	Bancroftian filariasis ('elephantiasis')	Ivermectin, DEC
Onchocerca volvulus	Onchocerciasis ('river blindness')	Ivermectin, DEC
Loa loa	Loaiasis ('eyeworm')	Ivermectin, DEC
Cestodes (tapeworms)		
Taenia saginata	Taeniasis (beef tapeworm)	Praziquantil, niclosamide
Taenia solium	Cysticercosis (pork tapeworm)	Praziquantil, niclosamide
Echinococcus granulosus	Echinococcosis, hydatidosis, hydatid cyst (dog tapeworm)	Albendazole and surgical removal of cysts
Trematodes (flukes)		
Schistosoma spp.	Schistosomiasis ('bilharzia')	Praziquantel
Fasciola hepatica	Fascioliasis	Bithionol

45   Non-drug control of infection

Infectious disease is an area in which pharmaceutical medicines allow treatment with eradication of the disease rather than mere palliation which occurs with other common disorders such as rheumatic and cardiovascular diseases. In the developing world, pharmaceutical medicines have prohibitive costs, and alternative remedies are used. Even in developed countries, when diseases are chronic or recurrent, alternative remedies may have a role as adjunctive or replacement therapy. Some infections are, in any case, already difficult to treat with known antibiotics, and others are due to organisms that have become resistant, such as VRE, MRSA and VRSA. Common colds are the commonest infections for which non-prescription medicines are taken: most treatments are for symptomatic relief only, but vitamin C and zinc tablets have been used in an attempt to treat or prevent the infection. The practice of evidence-based medicine is being applied to these forms of therapy.

Psychotherapy The science of **psychoneuroimmunology** has shown that the systems of the body do not work in isolation. Psychological status, and moods, have been shown to have effects on the immune system, possibly via neural and endocrine networks. There is good evidence that a positive emotional outlook leads to lower frequency and severity of common colds irrespective of other known risk factors. Supporting this is the finding that these same people have an enhanced cell-mediated immunity. Decades ago, psychotherapy was described in the medical literature as successful therapy for common colds but was not pursued. Use of psychological manipulation is now used for control of recurrent infections, such as genital herpes, with reported success, but has yet to be fully evaluated in case-controlled studies. Similarly, there needs to be a full evaluation of the role of mood on vaccine response, as there is a suggestion that a positive mood enhances it.

Herbal and 'natural' remedies In the developing world there are many 'natural therapies' used to treat infections. Even in Europe it is estimated that the herbal remedy market is worth £1.5 billion, with herbal remedies being freely available for public consumption. The use of plant-derived remedies in allopathic medicine is also well established; digoxin derived from the *Digitalis* plant is a well-known example. A standard therapy for warts has been podophyllin from the herb *Podophyllum peltatum*. Artemeter and sodium artenusate (new treatments for malaria) have been derived from artemisin, a natural product from *Artemesia annua* used as a herbal remedy for centuries. *Phyllanthrus amarus*, duckweed plant, has been the source of a remedy for jaundice in Asia for centuries; case-control studies of its use for treating chronic hepatitis B have shown benefit and offer prospects for the treatment for a disease that is not well-managed by currently licensed drugs. A component of chilli peppers, capsaicin, has antiviral properties but is now used in herpes zoster infections because of its ability to control zoster-associated pain. There are many pharmaceutical companies now exploring this area of **phytopharmacy**, also known as **ethnobotany** if based on traditional remedies. Evaluation and control of such therapies is likely to be subject to the same stringency as other drugs, with the recognition that such treatments are not without side effects.

Other strategies Many viruses are temperature sensitive and do not replicate outside a defined range. This has been exploited for the treatment of common colds, as the two commonest causes, rhinoviruses and coronaviruses, replicate best at 33°C. Devices that raise the temperature inside the nose to above 35°C abort replication. Unfortunately for this approach, there are other viruses that cause the common cold which replicate well at the higher temperature.

Controlling bacteria–bacteria communication, which occurs through substances known as homoserine lactones, is a strategy that is under exploration. This approach may have the inherent advantage, if successful, of encouraging pathogens to be commensals and beneficial. Natural antimicrobial peptides from insects, plants and animals are also under investigation in an era where resistance to known antibiotics is on the increase and the rising cost of development of new drugs is commercially prohibitive for the pharmaceutical companies.

The principles of evidence-based medicine have not been applied to the use of other approaches, such as homeopathy and acupuncture, or if applied have not yet shown benefit.

Genetically modified micro-organisms (GMOS) in the environment and biotechnology

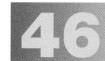

Micro-organisms should not be viewed solely as harmful, as many of them fulfil vital roles in our industrialised society (**Table 46.1**). The process of continuously selecting yeast strains that produce the best bread or beer is an example of how the genes of micro-organisms have been modified as part of a 'natural' process, but the possibilities (and concerns) have increased enormously with recent advances in **genetic engineering**. The principal problem then is trying to predict how an organism will behave with a gene that has never existed in that environment before and how to ensure that the novel gene cannot spread any further to other micro-organisms.

GMOs in the laboratory The use of antibiotics encourages antibiotic-resistant organisms, including those that arise through mutation. Clinical laboratories will grow these strains up to large numbers from patient samples as part of the diagnostic process, but their working practices are controlled by strict guidelines to prevent the spread of infections. Similar restrictions are placed upon research laboratories that may purposely create hybrid strains of pathogens through **gene cloning** for the study of pathogenesis or vaccine production; here, a gene of interest is transferred into a 'laboratory' bacterium where it may be easier to study its activity, where it is simpler to generate and monitor the effects of gene mutation, and where it may be possible to produce much larger amounts of the factor of interest than in the 'wild' strain.

GMOs in humans/animals There is a long history of giving GMOs to humans and animals through the process of immunisation. However, this movement is now more focused because of molecular biology, with engineered vaccines planned for many infectious diseases (e.g. Hepatitis B, *H. influenzae* b) and also some tumours (e.g. cervical carcinoma, malignant melanoma). In addition, some engineered viruses (e.g. adenovirus and canary pox) will probably be used as vectors during **gene therapy**, for example in cystic fibrosis, delivering a fully functional copy of the *cftr* gene to the affected individual. There is also some concern that mutated or hybrid micro-organisms might arise accidentally as a result of **xenotransplantation**: an animal pathogen might be transferred along with the donor organ. Particularly as the host would be deliberately immunosuppressed, there might be sufficient time for the agent to multiply and adapt to the human host, with implications then for the entire population.

GMOs in the environment There are now over forty separate microbial 'biocontrol' agents available for use as pesticides, some with a history of use going back to the 1940s. This area is likely to expand with the development of genetically engineered plants and other microbes for industrial uses. Controls on this work are in place as there are a number of potential concerns, as yet unproven:

- Some of these products were generated using bacterial host/vector systems which include the use of antibiotic resistance genes as selectable markers during cloning. As these resistance genes were not subsequently removed, there is a risk of increased spread of antibiotic resistance.

- These novel products are introduced into an environment in which they may not normally be found, and therefore the effects are somewhat unpredictable. They may have a deleterious effect on the homeostasis of that environment themselves, or some of their DNA may be taken up into other organisms, with unknown consequences.

- Humans might be exposed to greater levels of these agents than previously. Should a problem arise, it is most likely to be one of allergy, but some of these agents could potentially act as pathogens. For example, *Burkholderia* (*Pseudomonas*) *cepacia* type Winconsin is currently used agriculturally for 'damping-off' disease in some countries, and some strains of this species are known to be an infective problem in patients with cystic fibrosis.

TABLE 46.1		
Microbiology in biotechnology		
Food/drug production		
• 'Traditional' foods	Cheese, yoghurt, wine, beer, bread and other fermented products	
• Protein supplements	Fungi, *Spirulina*	
• Antibiotics	*Streptomyces*, *Bacillus*, fungi	
• Organic acid production	e.g. acetic acid, citric acid	
• Complex steroid production		
• Amino acid production	e.g. monosodium glutamate	
• Bacterial enzymes	Biological detergents, diagnostic reagents	
Environmental effects		
• Insect control	*Bacillus thuringiensis*, cytoplasmic polyhedrosis viruses	
• Biohydrometallergy	Leach pile mining of copper	
• Bioremediation	Oil spill degradation, sewage treatment	

47 Immunisation to infectious disease

When Edward Jenner demonstrated, in 1796, that inoculation with material from cowpox-infected tissue could protect against subsequent exposure to smallpox, the science of **immunisation** was born; preparations that induce immunity are now commonly known as **vaccines**, derived from the name of the cowpox agent (the **vaccinia** virus). Vaccines are important against diseases that may have serious consequences and where treatments are less than optimal, particularly when infection is common. **Fig. 47.1** shows how effective they can be: the decline in cases of whooping cough coincided with the introduction of the pertussis vaccine in the 1950s, but notifications rose again when fears over safety of the vaccine led to decreased uptake in the 1970s.

Adaptive immunity may be produced by two methods:

- **Passive immunisation** produces immunity by giving preparations of specific antibody collected from individuals convalescing from infection or post-immunisation, or human normal immunoglobulin from pooled blood donor plasma if the infectious agent is prevalent (**Table 47.1**).
- **Active immunisation** involves the administration of vaccines to induce a response from the host's own immune system. It is the most powerful method, effective against a wide range of pathogens (**Appendix 8**, p. 132) and, as in most parts of the world, now used routinely in the UK (**Table 47.2**).

Vaccine design

Historically, vaccines have been produced by **inactivating** the infectious agent or else **attenuating** it by multiple passage through a non-human host. Some work via a Th2-type response to stimulate the production of antibody, for example against the pathogen's adhesins or toxin-binding regions; even the low levels of antibody found years later are sufficient either to abort the infection or prevent severe disease; in this context, it may be particularly important to induce mucosal antibody. Vaccines that increase cell-mediated immunity promote a Th1-type response, producing memory T cells that will respond more rapidly and effectively on subsequent exposure to the pathogen. Many vaccines require oily **adjuvants** that non-specifically boost the immune response at the injection site. However, now that more is understood about the way that vaccines work, those currently under development will be engineered using molecular biological techniques so that they direct the immune response in the manner appropriate to each agent; they should be more immunogenic, have fewer side effects and be less likely to revert to the harmful wild type than traditional vaccines. Simple DNA vaccines are effective because the host cell takes up free DNA, expresses it and so induces an immune response against the foreign protein(s).

Problems with vaccines

The **adverse effects** that might be expected after immunisation depend on which vaccine was given, but local pain and inflammation, headache, malaise and temperature (even febrile convulsions) are reasonably common. Serious problems, such as encephalopathy, are extremely rare and certainly less than the morbidity/mortality that might be expected from natural infection. Contrary to popular belief, there are few **contra-indications** to vaccination: it is not recommended for those with a significant acute infection or with hypersensitivity to the same vaccine previously; *some* live vaccines are contra-indicated in the immunocompromised, almost all in the pregnant. Very rarely, a vaccine such as oral polio will revert back towards the wild virus and may cause disease in susceptible contacts. Whilst the goal of immunisation is the protection of the vaccinated, it also has implications for the whole population (**Fig. 47.2**). If immunisation produces high levels of **herd immunity** (case A), infection cannot spread, and a small number of susceptible individuals will be safe; if herd immunity is maintained by global immunisation together with case isolation, a solely human virulent pathogen may be eradicated, as happened with smallpox. As the number of vaccine failures/refusers slowly builds up (case B → C → D), a critical point is reached when infection can again spread widely. However, many susceptible individuals will now be relatively old, and therefore the frequency of severe complications is much increased compared with the pattern of disease prior to the introduction of vaccination. The quality control of vaccine production must be flawless; if a pathogen is incompletely inactivated or a vaccine becomes contaminated, the consequences may be disastrous.

TABLE 47.1

The use of passive immunisation

Preparation	Use
Hyperimmune immunoglobulin	Post-exposure prophylaxis against: <ul><li>tetanus</li><li>hepatitis B</li><li>diphtheria</li><li>rabies</li><li>chickenpox (immunocompromised only)</li></ul>
Human normal deficiency immunoglobulin	<ul><li>regular administration if severe antibody</li><li>pre-exposure prophylaxis against hepatitis A in travellers to endemic regions</li><li>post-exposure prophylaxis against measles (immunocompromised) or rubella (susceptible pregnant)</li></ul>

TABLE 47.2

The UK immunisation schedule

Vaccine	Age
Diphtheria/tetanus/pertussis (DTP) & *H. influenzae* b (Hib); polio	2 months 3 months 4 months
Measles/mumps/rubella (MMR)	12–15 months
Booster diphtheria/tetanus (DT); polio; 2nd dose measles/mumps/rubella	3–5 years
BCG (against *M. tuberculosis*)	10–14 years
Booster diphtheria/tetanus; polio	13–18 years

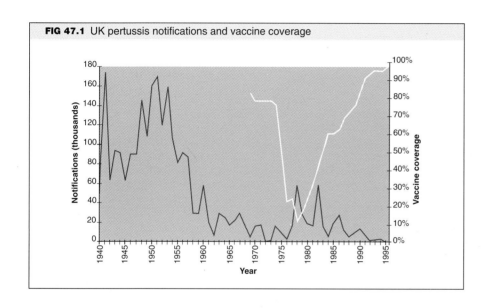

FIG 47.1 UK pertussis notifications and vaccine coverage

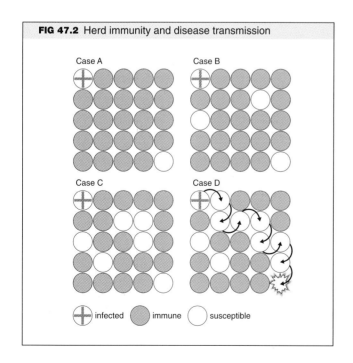

FIG 47.2 Herd immunity and disease transmission

Case A Case B Case C Case D

⊕ infected ⬤ immune ◯ susceptible

Appendices

APPENDIX
1

Answers

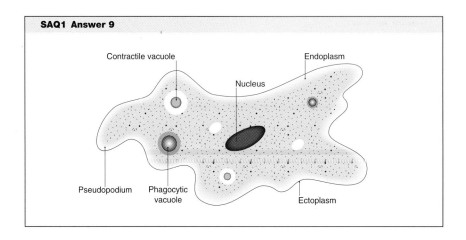

SAQ1 Answer 9

- Contractile vacuole
- Nucleus
- Endoplasm
- Pseudopodium
- Phagocytic vacuole
- Ectoplasm

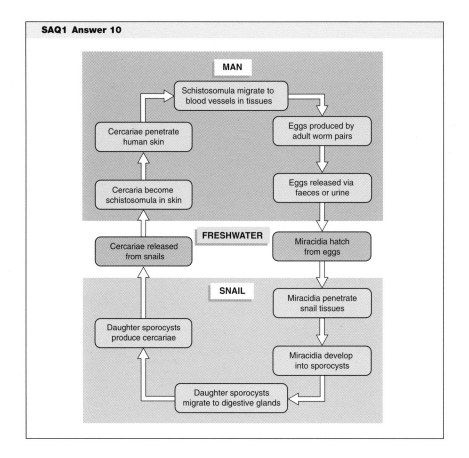

SAQ1 Answer 10

MAN

Schistosomula migrate to blood vessels in tissues

Cercariae penetrate human skin

Eggs produced by adult worm pairs

Cercaria become schistosomula in skin

Eggs released via faeces or urine

FRESHWATER

Cercariae released from snails

Miracidia hatch from eggs

SNAIL

Daughter sporocysts produce cercariae

Miracidia penetrate snail tissues

Miracidia develop into sporocysts

Daughter sporocysts migrate to digestive glands

SAQ2 Answer 8

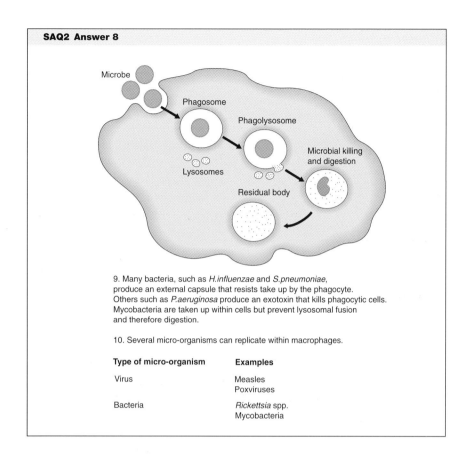

9. Many bacteria, such as *H.influenzae* and *S.pneumoniae*, produce an external capsule that resists take up by the phagocyte. Others such as *P.aeruginosa* produce an exotoxin that kills phagocytic cells. Mycobacteria are taken up within cells but prevent lysosomal fusion and therefore digestion.

10. Several micro-organisms can replicate within macrophages.

Type of micro-organism	Examples
Virus	Measles
	Poxviruses
Bacteria	*Rickettsia* spp.
	Mycobacteria

CS3 Answer 6 Pathogenesis of endotoxic shock

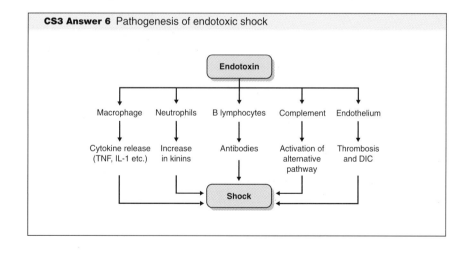

The language of microbiology

Below is a list of some terms commonly used in medical microbiology.

acid-fast Bacteria retaining initial stain and difficult to decolorise with acid alcohol.

aerobe Any oxygen-requiring organism. Compare **anaerobe**.

aetiology The study of the cause of a disease.

agar A dried polysaccharide extract of seaweed used as a solidifying agent in microbiological media.

anaerobe An organism that grows in the absence of molecular oxygen. Compare **aerobe**.

antagonism The killing, injury, or inhibition of growth of one species of micro-organism by another when one organism adversely affects the environment of the other.

antibiotic A substance of microbial origin that has antimicrobial activity.

antimicrobial agent Any chemical or biological agent that destroys or inhibits growth of micro-organisms.

antiseptic A disinfectant that can be applied to the skin to prevent or stop growth of micro-organisms.

antitoxin An antibody capable of uniting with and neutralising a specific toxin.

arthropod An invertebrate with jointed legs, such as an insect or a crustacean.

asepsis A condition in which harmful micro-organisms are absent.

aseptic technique Precautionary measures taken to prevent contamination.

asymptomatic Exhibiting no symptoms.

attenuation Weakening; reduction in virulence.

autoclave An apparatus using steam under pressure for sterilisation.

bacillus Any rod-shaped bacterium.

bacteraemia A condition in which bacteria are present in the bloodstream.

bactericide. An agent that destroys bacteria.

bacteriophage A virus that infects bacteria and causes lysis of bacterial cells.

bacteriostasis Inhibition of growth and reproduction of bacteria without killing them.

bacterium, pl. **bacteria** Diverse and ubiquitous prokaryotic single-celled micro-organism.

beta haemolysis A colourless, defined zone of haemolysis surrounding certain bacterial colonies growing on blood agar.

capsule An envelope or slime layer surrounding the cell wall of certain micro-organisms.

carrier A person in apparently good health who harbours a pathogenic micro-organism.

chancre The primary ulcerative lesion in syphilis.

chemotaxis Movement of an organism in response to a chemical stimulus.

chemotherapy Treatment of disease by the use of chemicals.

cilium, pl. **cilia** A hair-like appendage on certain cells.

clone A population of cells descended from a single cell.

coagulase An enzyme, produced by pathogenic staphylococci, that causes coagulation of blood plasma.

coccus A spherical bacterium.

colony A macroscopically visible growth of micro-organisms on a solid culture medium.

commensalism A relationship between members of different species living in proximity in which one organism benefits from the association but the other is not affected.

compromised host A person already weakened with debilitating disease.

conjugation A mating process characterised by the temporary fusion of the mating partners and transfer of genes. Conjugation occurs particularly in unicellular organisms.

contamination Entry of undesirable organisms into some material or object.

culture A population of micro-organisms cultivated in a medium.

decimal reduction time The time required to reduce a viable microbial population by 90%. Usually applied to heat or chemical disinfection.

denature The modification, by physical or chemical action, of the structure of an organic substance (e.g. protein) in order to alter some properties of the substance, such as solubility.

dimorphism Occurring in two forms.

disease A state of impaired body function occurring as a response to infection, stress, or other conditions.

disinfectant An agent that kills most, but not all, micro-organisms.

DNA polymerase An enzyme that adds nucleotides and synthesises DNA in one direction.

dysentery Disease due to infection of the lower intestine.

endemic Peculiar to or occurring constantly in a community.

endogenous Produced or originating from within.

endotoxin A toxin produced in an organism and liberated only when the organism disintegrates.

enteric Pertaining to the intestines.

enteropathogen An organism that causes intestinal disease.

enterotoxin A toxin specific for cells of the intestine. It gives rise to symptoms of food poisoning.

epidemic A sudden increase in the incidence of a disease, affecting large numbers of people over a wide area.

epidemiology The study of the factors that influence the occurrence and distribution of disease in groups of individuals.

eukaryote A cell that possesses a definitive or true nucleus. Compare **prokaryote**.

exogenous Produced or originating from without.

exospore A spore external to the vegetative cell.

exotoxin A toxin excreted by a micro-organism into the surrounding medium.

F factor The fertility or sex factor in the cytoplasm of male bacterial cells.

fibrinolysin A substance, produced by haemolytic streptococci, that can liquefy clotted blood plasma or fibrin clots. Also called **streptokinase**.

fimbriae, sing. **fimbria** Surface appendages of certain Gram-negative bacteria composed of protein subunits. Also called **pili**.

fission An asexual process by which some micro-organisms reproduce.

flagellates One of the subphyla of the Phylum *Protozoa*.

flagellum, pl. **flagella** Whip-like appendage on cells used for locomotion.

flora In microbiology, the micro-organisms present in a given situation, e.g. intestinal flora.

fomite A non-food substance or surface that is able to be a source of infection, e.g. clothing.

fulminating infection A sudden, severe and rapidly progressing infectious disease.

fungicide An agent that kills or destroys fungi.

gamete A reproductive cell that fuses with another reproductive cell to form a zygote, which then develops into a new individual; a sex cell.

gastroenteritis Inflammation of the mucosa of the stomach and intestine.

generation time The time interval necessary for a cell to divide.

genotype The particular set of genes present in an organism and its cells; an organism's genetic constitution. Compare **phenotype**.

genus, pl. **genera** A group of very closely related species.

germicide An agent capable of killing germs, usually pathogenic micro-organisms.

Gram-negative bacteria Bacteria that appear red after being subjected to the Gram stain.

Gram-positive bacteria Bacteria that appear blue or violet after being subjected to the Gram stain.

Gram stain A differential stain by which bacteria are classed as Gram-positive or Gram-negative depending upon whether they retain or lose the primary stain (crystal violet when subjected to treatment with a decolorising agent).

H antigen A type of antigen found in the flagella of certain bacteria.

haemolysis The process of dissolving red blood cells.

host An organism harbouring another as a parasite or infectious agent.

ID Infective dose; the number of micro-organisms required to infect a host.

ID$_{50}$ The dose (number of micro-organisms) that will infect 50% of the experimental animals in a test series.

incubation In microbiology, the subjecting of cultures of micro-organisms to conditions (especially temperatures) favourable to their growth.

infectious Capable of producing disease in a susceptible host.

inoculation The artificial introduction of micro-organisms or substances into the body or into a culture medium.

inoculum The substance, containing micro-organisms or other material, that is introduced in inoculation.

in vitro Literally, 'in glass' and pertaining to biological experiments performed in test tubes or other laboratory vessels. Compare **in vivo**.

in vivo Within the living organism; pertaining to laboratory testing of agents within living organisms. Compare **in vitro**.

Koch's postulates Guidelines to prove that a disease is caused by a specific micro-organism.

LD$_{50}$ The dose (number of micro-organisms) that will kill 50% of the animals in a test series.

morphology The branch of biological science that deals with the study of the structure and form of living organisms.

mycology The study of fungi.

mycoplasma A group of bacteria composed of highly pleomorphic cells.

mycosis A disease caused by fungi.

mycotoxin Any toxic substance produced by fungi.

nosocomial disease. Describing or pertaining to disease acquired in the hospital.

oedema Excessive accumulation of fluid in body tissue.

opportunistic micro-organism A micro-organism that exists as part of the normal microbiota (flora) but becomes pathogenic when transferred from the normal habitat into other areas of the host or when host resistance is lowered.

pandemic A world-wide epidemic.

parasite An organism that derives its nourishment from a living plant or animal host. A parasite does not necessarily cause disease.

parasitism The relationship of a parasite to its host.

parenteral By some route other than via the intestinal tract.

pasteurisation The process of heating liquid food or beverage at a controlled temperature to enhance the keeping quality and destroy harmful micro-organisms.

pathogen An organism capable of producing disease.

peritrichous Having flagella around the entire surface of the cell.

phage See **bacteriophage**.

phage-typing Identifying a pathogenic bacterium by the pattern of lysis caused by different phage-types.

phenotype The observable characteristics of an organism. Compare **genotype**.

phylogeny The evolutionary or ancestral history of organisms.

phylum, pl. **phyla** A taxon consisting of a group of related classes.

pilus See **fimbriae**.

potable Suitable for drinking.

prokaryote A type of cell in which the nuclear substance is not enclosed within a membrane: e.g. a bacterium. Compare **eukaryote**.

prophylaxis Preventive treatment for protection against disease.

protist A micro-organism in the kingdom *Protista*.

protozoa Single-celled eukaryotic micro-organisms.

protozoology The study of protozoa.

pseudopodium A temporary projection of the protoplast of an amoeboid cell in which cytoplasm flows during extension and withdrawal.

resistance-transfer factor A factor that confers on micro-organisms resistance to a number of antibiotics. Abbreviation: R factor.

rickettsia Obligate intracellular bacteria of arthropods, many types of which are pathogenic for humans and other mammals.

sanitiser An agent that reduces the microbial flora in materials or on such articles as eating utensils to levels judged safe by public health authorities

saprophyte An organism living on dead organic matter.

schizogony Asexual reproduction by multiple fission of a trophozoite (a vegetative protozoan).

schizont A stage in the asexual life cycle of the malaria parasites.

septicaemia A systemic disease caused by the invasion and multiplication of pathogenic micro-organisms in the blood-stream.

sequela A complication following a disease.

species A single kind of micro-organism; a subdivision of a genus.

spirochete A spiral form of bacterium; most are parasitic.

spore A resistant body formed by certain micro-organisms; a resistant resting cell; a primitive unicellular dormant body.

sporicide An agent that kills spores.

sporozoite A motile infective stage of certain sporozoans, resulting from sexual reproduction, that gives rise to an asexual cycle in a new host.

staphylococci Spherical bacteria (cocci) occurring in irregular, grape-like clusters.

sterile Free of living organisms.

sterilisation The process of making sterile by killing all forms of life.

stock cultures Known species of micro-organisms maintained in the laboratory for various tests and studies.

strain A pure culture of micro-organisms composed of the descendants of a single isolation.

streptococci Cocci that divide in such a way that chains of cells are formed.

susceptibility The state of being open to disease; specifically, capability of being infected; lack of immunity.

symbiosis The living together of two or more organisms; microbial association.

syndrome A group of signs and symptoms that characterises a disease.

systematics The science of animal, plant and microbial classification.

taxis Movement away from or toward a chemical substance or physical condition.

taxonomy The science of classification of organisms, usually based on natural relationships.

teichoic acid A cell-wall constituent unique to prokaryotes.

thermolabile Destroyed by heat at temperatures below 100°C.

thermostable Resistant to temperatures of 100°C.

tissue culture A growth of tissue cells **in vitro** in a laboratory medium.

topical application Application to a localised area.

toxin A poisonous substance elaborated by an organism, such as a bacterial toxin.

trophozoite The vegetative form of a protozoan.

tuberculin An extract of the tuberculosis bacilli capable of eliciting an inflammatory reaction in an animal body that has been sensitised by the presence of living or dead tubercle bacilli. Used in a skin test for tuberculosis.

vaccination Inoculation with a biologic preparation (a vaccine) to produce immunity.

vaccine A suspension of disease-producing micro-organisms modified by killing or attenuation so that it will not cause disease and can stimulate the formation of antibodies upon inoculation.

vector An agent, such as an insect, capable of mechanically or biologically transferring a pathogen from one organism to another.

vegetative stage The stage of active growth, as opposed to the resting or spore stages.

viable Capable of living, growing and developing; alive.

viraemia The presence of virus in the blood.

viricide An agent that kills viruses.

virology The study of viruses.

virulence The capacity of a micro-organism to produce disease; pathogenicity.

virus An obligate intracellular parasitic micro-organism that is smaller than bacteria.

yeast A kind of fungus that is unicellular and not characterised by typical mycelia.

zoonosis Animal disease transmissible to human beings.

Commonly used abbreviations

As with all branches of medicine, abbreviations are routinely used in medical microbiology where they provide a convenient 'shorthand' for describing laboratory and clinical findings. However, abbreviations should be used cautiously as they may be employed in another branch of medicine to describe a totally different test or clinical finding. Below is a list of some common medical microbiology abbreviations.

AAFB	acid-alcohol-fast bacilli
AFB	acid-fast bacilli
AHG	anti-human globulin (antibodies, serum)
AIDS	acquired immune deficiency syndrome
ASO	antistreptolysin O
ATS	anti-tetanus serum
BCG	Bacille Calmette–Guérin
C1, C2 etc.	complement components
cAMP	cyclic adenosine monophosphate
CAPD	Continuous ambulatory peritoneal dialysis
CFT	complement-fixation test
cfu	colony-forming unit
CIE	countercurrent immunoelectrophoresis
CJD	Creutzfeld–Jakob disease
CMV	cytomegalovirus
CNS	central nervous system
CPE	cytopathic effect
CSF	cerebrospinal fluid
CSU	catheter specimen of urine
CTL	cytotoxic T lymphocyte
DEAFF	detection of early antigen fluorescent foci (used for diagnosis of CMV)
DNA	deoxyribonucleic acid
DPT	diphtheria, pertussis, tetanus combined (triple) vaccine
EBV	Epstein–Barr virus
ECHO	enteric cytopathic human orphan (viruses)
ELISA	enzyme-linked immunosorbent assay
EMU	early morning urine (specimen of)
EPEC	enteropathogenic *Escherichia coli*
ETEC	enterotoxigenic *Escherichia coli*
Fab, Fc	antibody-binding (ab) and complement-binding (c) parts of immunoglobulin molecule
FTA	fluorescent treponemal antibody (test)
GALT	gut-associated lymphoid tissue
GC	gonococcus

GC ratio	guanidine + cytosine mol. % content of DNA
GCFT	gonococcal complement-fixation test
GLC	gas-liquid chromatography
HAI	haemagglutination-inhibition (test)
HBsAg etc.	antigenic components of hepatitis B virus
Hib	*Haemophilus influenzae* type b
HIV	human immunodeficiency virus (AIDS associated)
HPV	human papilloma virus
HSV	herpes simplex virus
HTLV	human T cell lymphotropic virus
HUS	haemolytic uraemic syndrome
HVS	high vaginal swab
ID	infective dose
IFN	interferon
IgA, IgE, etc.	immunoglobulins of classes, A, E, etc.
IL	interleukin
IM	intramuscular
INAH	isonicotinic acid hydrazide isoniazid
IPV	inactivated polio vaccine
i.v. or IV	intravenous
K	capsular or envelope (antigens, antibodies)
LCR	Ligase chain reaction
LD_{50}	dose lethal to 50% of a group of experimental animals
LF	lactose-fermenter
LGV	lymphogranuloma venereum
LPS	lipopolysaccharide
LRTI	Lower respiratory tract infection
LT	heat-labile toxin (of *Escherichia coli*)
Mab	monoclonal antibody
MBC	minimal bactericidal concentration
MIC	minimal inhibitory concentration
MIC_{90}	concentration that inhibits 90% of a group of bacterial strains
MIF	macrophage-migration-inhibiting factor

MLD	minimum lethal dose (of a drug or microbial preparation)	**TAB (TABC)**	typhoid + paratyphoids A and B (and C) vaccine
MMR	measles, mumps, rubella (vaccine)	**TB**	tubercle bacilli (used to denote tuberculosis)
MRSA	methicillin (multi-) resistant *Staphylococcus aureus*	**TCID**	tissue culture infective dose
MSU	mid-stream urine (specimen of)	**TNF**	tumour necrosis factor
		TORCH	toxoplasma, rubella virus, cytomegalovirus, herpes simplex virus (acronym for four infectious agents that must be considered in congenital infections)
NGU	non-gonococcal urethritis		
NLF	non-lactose-fermenter		
NK	natural killer (cell)		
NSU	non-specific urethritis	**TPHA**	*Treponema pallidum* haemagglutination (test)
NSV	non-specific vaginitis (anaerobic vaginosis)	**TPI**	*Treponema pallidum* immobilisation (test)
		TRIC	trachoma and inclusion conjunctivitis (agents)
OPV	oral polio vaccine	**TT**	(1) tetanus toxoid (2) tuberculin tested (cattle)
PABA	p-aminobenzoic acid		
PCR	polymerase chain reaction		
pfu	plaque-forming unit	**UHT**	ultra-heat treated (milk)
PGU	post-gonococcal urethritis	**URTI**	upper respiratory tract infection
PMC	pseudomembranous colitis	**UTI**	urinary tract infection
PPD	purified protein derivative (of old tuberculin)		
		VDRL	Venereal Diseases Research Laboratory (test)
psi	pounds per square inch		
PUO	pyrexia of unknown origin	**Vi**	virulence (antigen of *Salmonella typhi*, etc.)
RIA	radioimmunoassay	**VRE**	vancomycin-resistant enterococci
RNA	ribonucleic acid	**VT**	vero cell cytotoxin (of *Escherichia coli*)
RS	respiratory syncytial (virus)		
		VTEC	verotoxigenic *Escherichia coli*
SDD	selective decontamination of the digestive tract	**VZ**	varicella-zoster (virus)
SPEAR	specific parenteral and enteral antiseptic regimen	**WR**	Wassermann reaction
spp.	species	**ZN**	Ziehl–Neelsen (staining method used to detect mycobacteria)
SSPE	subacute sclerosing panencephalitis		

Notifiable diseases (UK)

In the UK, many infections are notifiable by law to the Consultant in Communicable Diseases Control or other appropriate officer:

- Acute encephalitis (not Scotland)
- Anthrax
- Chickenpox (not England & Wales)
- Cholera
- Diphtheria
- Dysentery
- Food poisoning (or suspected in England & Wales)
- Gastroenteritis (if under 2 years of age, Northern Ireland only)
- Lassa fever (separate category in England & Wales only)
- Legionellosis (not England & Wales)
- Leprosy (not Northern Ireland)
- Leptospirosis
- Malaria
- Measles
- Meningitis ('acute' only in Northern Ireland)
- Meningococcal septicaemia without meningitis (only England & Wales)
- Mumps
- Ophthalmia neonatorum (only England & Wales)
- Paratyphoid fever
- Plague
- Poliomyelitis
- Puerperal fever (Scotland only)
- Rabies
- Relapsing fever
- Rubella
- Scarlet fever (not Scotland)
- Smallpox
- Tetanus (not Scotland)
- Tuberculosis (not Scotland)
- Typhoid fever (not Scotland)
- Typhus
- Viral haemorrhagic fever
- Viral hepatitis
- Whooping cough
- Yellow fever (not Scotland).

Common helminth infections of humans

Organism	Disease and site of infection	Mode of transmission	Geographic distribution
Nematodes — worms			
Ancylostoma duodenalis	Old World hookworm: gut, lungs and heart; malnutrition, pneumonitis, anaemia	Larvae excreted into soil and infect through skin (usually foot)	Mediterranean, southern USA, S. America, Africa, Asia
Necator americanus	New World hookworm (symptoms as above)	Larvae excreted into soil and infect through skin (usually foot)	Southern USA, C. & S. America, Africa, Asia
Strongyloides stercoralis	Stronglyloidiasis (symptoms as for hookworms)	Larvae excreted into soil and infect through skin (usually foot)	As for hookworms
Ascaris lumbricoides	Ascariasis ('roundworm'): symptoms as for hookworms	Faecal-oral ingestion of eggs	Southern USA, C. & S. America, Africa, Asia, Australia
Toxocara canis (dog) and T. cati (cat)	Toxocariasis: visceral larval migrans (tissues), ocular larval migrans (eye)	Faecal-oral ingestion of eggs	World-wide
Trichuris trichiura	Trichuriasis: ('whipworm'): gut infection, malnutrition	Faecal-oral ingestion of eggs	As for Ascaris
Enterobius vermicularis	Enterobiasis: ('pinworm'): anal itching, diarrhoea	Faecal-oral ingestion of eggs	World-wide
Nematodes — filaria			
Wuchereria bancrofti	Bancroftian filariasis ('elephantiasis'): fever and lymphangitis leading to obstruction of the lymphatics	Insect vector: mosquitoes (Anopheles and Aedes)	South America, central Africa, Far East
Onchocerca volvulus	Onchocerciasis ('river blindness'): lymphadenopathy, in groin and axilla, intradermal oedema and pachyderma ('crocodile' skin), keratitis, retinochoroiditis	Insect vector: blackfly (Simulium)	C. America, C. Africa and the Yemen
Loa loa	Loaiasis ('eyeworm'): migration of worm in eyelid, vitreous and anterior chamber	Insect vector: mango flies (Chrysops)	Central and West Africa
Cestodes (tapeworms)			
Taenia saginata (beef tapeworm)	Taeniasis: asymptomatic or abdominal pain, diarrhoea, weight loss	Ingestion of infected beef	World-wide
Taenia solium (pork tapeworm)	Cysticercosis: larvae penetrate gut and form cysticerci in muscles	Ingestion of infected pork	South and central America, China, Indonesia
Echinococcus granulosus (dog tapeworm)	Echinococcosis, hydatidosis, hydatid cyst infection of liver	Faecal-oral ingestion of eggs from dogs	World-wide
Trematodes (flukes)			
Schistosoma species	Schistosomiasis ('bilharzia'): liver, bladder (S. haematobium) and rectum (S. mansoni, S. japonicum)	Cercariae from snail cycle burrow into skin when standing in water	South America, West Indies, Africa, Middle East, Egypt, Far East
Fasciola hepatica	Fascioliasis: fever, hepatomegaly, jaundice, bile duct obstruction	Ingestion of metacercariae from snail host	World-wide

Newly emerging pathogens and diseases

Year	Pathogen	Disease
1973	Rotavirus	Infantile diarrhoea
1975	Parvovirus B19	Aplastic crisis; fetal loss
1976	*Cryptosporidium*	Acute and chronic diarrhoea
1977	Ebola virus	Haemorrhagic fever
1977	*Legionella pneumophila*	Legionnaire's disease
1977	Hantaan virus	Haemorrhagic fever and renal syndrome
1977	*Campylobacter jejuni*	Diarrhoea
1980	Human T lymphotropic virus I (HTLV-I)	T cell lymphoma
1981	Toxin (TSST-1) producing *Staphylococcus aureus*	Toxic shock syndrome
1982	*Escherichia coli* O157:H7	Haemorrhagic colitis; haemolytic uraemic syndrome
1982	Human T lymphotropic virus II (HTLV-II)	Hairy cell leukaemia
1982	*Borrelia burgdorferi* and related species	Lyme disease
1983	Human immunodeficiency virus (HIV)	Acquired immunodeficiency syndrome (AIDS)
1983	*Helicobacter pylori*	Peptic ulcer disease; gastric carcinoma
1984	*Haemophilus influenzae* bio. Aegyptius	Brazilian purpuric fever
1985	*Enterocytozoon bieneusi*	Persistent diarrhoea
1986	*Cyclospora cayetanensis*	Persistent diarrhoea
1986	Human immunodeficiency virus 2 (HIV-2)	AIDS
1988	Human herpesvirus 6 (HHV6)	Roseola subitum
1988	Hepatitis E	Enterally transmitted hepatitis
1989	Hepatitis C	Parenterally transmitted hepatitis
1989	*Ehrlichia chafeensis*	Human ehrlichiosis
1991	Guanarito virus	Venezuelan haemorrhagic fever
1991	*Encephalitozoon hellem*	Conjunctivitis, disseminated disease
1991	New species of *Babesia*	Atypical babesiosis
1991	*Tropheryma whippelii*	Whipple's disease
1992	*Vibrio cholerae* O139	Cholera
1992	*Bartonella henselae*	Cat scratch fever; bacillary angiomatosis
1993	Sin Nombre virus	Adult respiratory distress syndrome
1994	Sabia virus	Brazilian haemorrhagic fever
1995	Human herpes virus 8 (HHV8)	Kaposi Sarcoma in AIDS
1996	Bovine spongiform encephalopathy prion	Variant Creutzfeld–Jacob disease

Examples of common disinfectants and antiseptics

Disinfectant	Example	Bacteria				Fungi	Viruses	Properties and uses
		Gram-negative	Gram-positive	Myco-bacteria	Spores			
Phenolics	Soluble phenolics (Clearsol, Stericol, Izal)	±	+	+	−	+	−	Surface disinfection; laboratory discard jars
	Chloroxylenols (Dettol)	−	±	−	−	−	−	Antiseptic; inactivated by hard water and organic matter; can support growth of *Pseudomonas* bacteria
	Hexachlorophene (bisphenol: Ster-Zac)	−	+	−	−	−	−	Antiseptic powder or soap formulation; toxic to babies through skin absorption
Halogens	Chlorine solutions (bleach): sodium hypochlorite (Chloros, Domestos, Milton); chlorinated isocyanurates: (Presept, Haztab); chlorine dioxide	+	+	−	±	+	+	Disinfection of surfaces; laboratory discard jars; bathing and drinking water; infant feeding bottles; food preparation areas and equipment; corrosive to metals and inactivated by organic matter
	Iodine (in alcohol) and iodophores (organic complexes of iodine): providone-iodine (Betadine)	+	+	+	±	+	+	Antiseptic preparation of preoperative skin site and hand washing
Alcohols	70% ethanol or isopropanol	+	+	+	−	−	±	Antiseptic (usually with chlorhexidine); surface disinfection
Aldehydes	Formaldehyde/formalin	+	+	+	+	+	+	Fumigation of microbiology safety cabinets and rooms; highly irritant
	Glutaraldehyde (Asep, Cidex, Totacide)	+	+	+	±	+	+	Disinfectant for laboratory equipment and surgical instruments (e.g. endoscopes)
Biguanides	Chlorhexidine (Hibiscrub, Hibiclens)	−	+	−	−	+	−	Antiseptic: hand wash (operating theatres), wound cleansing, contact lens disinfection
Quaternary ammonium compounds	Cetrimide (with chlorhexidine: Savlon, Dettox)	±	+	−	−	±	−	Antiseptic: wound cleansing
	Benzalkonium chloride	±	+	−	−	+	−	Contact lens disinfection and preservative in skin creams
Others	Hydrogen peroxide	+	+	−	−	−	±	Contact lens disinfection, milk carton production
	Ultraviolet (UV) light	+	+	±	−	±	±	Water treatment
	Ozone	+	+	+	+	+	+	Water treatment

+, strong activity; −, little or no activity; ±, variable activity depending on organism type, or requires prolonged contact times

Vaccines available in the UK

Vaccine	Preparation	Additional comments
Diphtheria	Toxoid	UK immunisation schedule
Tetanus	Toxoid	UK immunisation schedule; post-exposure prophylaxis
Pertussis	Whole cell killed	UK immunisation schedule; acellular vaccines (pertussis toxin and haemagglutinin) becoming available
Haemophilus influenzae b	Capsular polysaccharide (conjugated)	UK immunisation schedule; asplenics
Polio	Live attenuated	UK immunisation schedule — oral (Sabin) in UK; inactivated injectable (Salk) also available
Measles	Live attenuated	UK immunisation schedule
Mumps	Live attenuated	UK immunisation schedule
Rubella	Live attenuated	UK immunisation schedule; women of child-bearing age with no evidence of immunity
BCG	Live attenuated	UK immunisation schedule
Anthrax	Toxin (enriched)	Only if risk of occupational exposure
Cholera	(Unavailable UK)	No longer recommended (WHO)
Hepatitis A	Inactivated	Travellers to endemic area; outbreaks; occupational risk; haemophiliacs and those with liver disease
Hepatitis B	Single protein	Neonates of positive mother; occupational risk; lifestyle; post-exposure prophylaxis
Influenza	Inactivated purified	Chronic respiratory disease; heart disease; renal failure; diabetes; immunosuppressed
Japanese encephalitis	Inactivated	Travellers to endemic area (unlicensed UK ⇒ 'named patient basis' only)
Meningococcal (groups A & C)	Purified polysaccharide	Travellers to endemic area; outbreaks; post-exposure prophylaxis; asplenic
Pneumococcal	Purified polysaccharide	As for influenza *plus* asplenics
Rabies	Inactivated	Occupational risk; post-exposure prophylaxis
Tick borne encephalitis	Inactivated	Travellers to endemic area (unlicensed UK ⇒ 'named patient basis' only)
Typhoid	Whole cell killed	Polysaccharide (Vi) and oral (Ty21a) vaccines now available: travellers to endemic area; occupational risk
Varicella zoster	Live attenuated	Immunocompromised (unlicensed UK ⇒ 'named patient basis' only)
Yellow fever	Live attenuated	Travellers (to endemic area or if vaccination certificate required for entry)

Further reading

This short book cannot fully do justice to the subject of infection. Most general medical textbooks have much more detail on the organisms, and review articles in medical and scientific journals will provide students with up-to-date comprehensive information on important infectious topics. There are also some specialist texts which can be 'dipped into' as supplemental reading for specific topics of interest:

Control of Communicable Diseases in Man. Benenson A (ed.). Mosby, St Louis.

Control of Hospital Infection. Ayliffe G A J et al (eds). Chapman & Hall, London.

Department of Health. Immunisation Against Infectious Disease. HMSO, London.

Medical Microbiology. Greenwood D, Slack R, Peutherer J (eds). Churchill Livingstone, Edinburgh.

Mims' Pathogenesis of Infectious disease. Mims C, Dimmock N, Nash A, Stephen J. Academic Press, London.

Microbiology. Davis B D, Dulbecco R, Eisen H N, Ginsberg H S. Lippincott, Philadelphia.

Principles and Practice of Infectious Disease. Mandell G L, Bennett J E, Dolin R (eds). Churchill Livingstone, New York.

Index

Abscesses
  amoebic liver, 84
  brain, 42–43
  breast, 62
  liver, 52, 84
  wound, 48
Aciclovir (acycloguanosine), 42, 46, 108
Acquired immunodeficiency syndrome
  (AIDS), 70–71
  see also Human immunodeficiency virus
Acute-phase proteins, 24
Adaptive immunity, 24, 26–27, 74, 75, 116
Adhesins, 6, 20, 54
Adhesion, 21
Adjuvants, 116
Aerobes, 6
Aflatoxin, 22
African trypanosomiasis (sleeping sickness),
  84, 86, 112
Air microbiology, 100
Airway infection, 36
Albendazole, 112
Alert organisms, 94
Allergies, 8, 9
Allyamines, 110
Amantadine, 34, 108
American trypanosomiasis
  (Chagas' disease), 64, 84, 86
Aminoglycosides, 102
Amoebae, 10, 11, 17
Amoebiasis, 84, 86, 112
Amoebic liver abscess, 84
Amoxicillin, 107
Amphixenoses, 76
Amphotericin B, 110, 112
Ampicillin, 102
Anaerobes, 6
Anaphylaxis, 102
Animal bites, 48
Anthropozoonoses, 76
Antibacterials (antibiotics), 2
  assays, 104
  case study, 106–107
  classes, 103
  diarrhoea, 50
  drug resistance, 90–91, 102
  overuse, 104
  pharmacology, 102
  principles, 102
  prophylaxis, 74, 104, 105
  resistance, 102, 107
  synergism, 104
  therapeutic index, 104
  therapy, 66–67, 104
  toxicity, 102
Antibiotics *see* Antibacterials
Antibodies *see* Immunoglobulins
Antibody-dependent cell cytotoxicity, 26
Antifungal therapy, 110–111
Antigen detection, 66
Antigen-presenting cells, 24
Antigenic drift/shift, 34
Antigenic variation, 29
Antigens, 26, 29
Antihelminthic therapy, 112, 113
Antimicrobial agents *see* Antibacterials
Antiprotozoal therapy, 112, 113
Antiretroviral drugs, 70
Antisense therapy, 108
Antiseptics, 98, 127
Antiviral therapy, 108
Apicomplexa, 10, 11
Apoptosis, 22
Arboviruses, 4
Archaea, 2

Artemeter, 114
Arthritis, 38, 64
Ascariasis (roundworm), 12, 13, 84, 87, 112
Aseptic technique, 94
Aspergillosis, 110
Aspergillus flavus, 22
Atovaquone, 72
Autoclaving, 98
Autoimmune diseases, 22–23
Azoles, 110

B cells (B lymphocytes), 26
Bacillus spp., 17
Bacillus stearothermophilis, 98
Bacteraemia, 54, 66, 69
Bacteria, 2, 3, 6, 17
  antibacterial resistance, 90–91, 102
  endocarditis, 54–55, 66
  Gram-stain reactions, 6, 7, 66–67
  growth rates, 7
  meningitis, 38, 39
  skin infections, 48–49
  tropical fevers, 84
Bacteriophages, 6
Bacteriuria, 56
Balantidiasis, 86
Bancroftian filariasis (elephantiasis),
  84, 87, 112
Bartonella henselae, 48, 90
Bell's palsy, 42
Benzimdazoles, 112
Benzofurans, 110
Benzylpenicillin, 41, 54, 102
Beta-hemolytic streptococci, 66
Bilharzia (schistosomiasis), 84, 87, 112
Biliary tract infections, 52
Binary fission, 6, 10
Biocides, 98
Biovars, 17
Bites, 48
Blackwater fever, 80, 83
Blepharitis, 44, 45
Blood-brain barrier, 38
Blood cultures, 30, 54, 66–67
Boils, 48
Bone infections, 64–65
Bone marrow, 26
  transplantation, 74
Bordetella pertussis infection
  (whooping cough), 36, 116
Borrelia spp., 6
Borrelia burgdorferi, 90
Botulism, 42
Brain
  abscess, 42–43
  biopsy, 42
Breast abscesses, 62
Bronchiolitis, 37
Bronchopneumonia, 36
Brucellosis, 84, 98
Bubonic plague, 85
Burkholderia (Pseudomonas) cepacia, 36
  type Wisconsin, 115

C-reactive proteins, 54
Calymmatobacterium granulomatis, 58
Campylobacter spp., 58, 74, 79, 90, 98
  enteritis, 42, 76
Candida albicans, 8
Candidiasis, 110
  skin, 48
  vaginal, 58, 61
Capsaicin, 114
Capsids, 4
Capsules, 20

Carbuncles, 48
Catheterisation, 56
Cefotaxime, 107
Ceftazidime, 107
Ceftriaxone, 41, 42, 107
Cefuroxime, 97, 102
Cellulitis, 48
  orbital, 44, 45
Cephalosporins, 36, 41, 56, 102, 107
Cerebrospinal fluid
  meningitis, 38, 39, 41
  viruses, 42
Cestodes (tapeworms), 12, 13, 64, 84, 87, 112
Chagas' disease, 64, 84, 86
Chancroid, 58
Chemotactic factors, 24
Chickenpox, 46
Chlamydia spp., 6, 17, 36, 62
Chlamydia trachomatis, 58, 61
Chloroquine, 80
Cholera, 84, 85
Choroid infections, 44, 45
Chromosomal mutation, 102
Chronic obstructive pulmonary disease
  (COPD), 36
Chronic renal failure, 74
Ciliates, 10, 11
Ciliophora, 10
Ciprofloxacin, 41, 61, 102, 107
Clades, 70
Clostridium spp., 17
Clostridium difficile, 50, 94, 102
Clotrimazole, 110
Cluster differentiation (CD), 26
Coagulases, 20
Coliforms, 66
Commensals, 2, 6, 8, 10, 50
Common colds, 34, 114
Complement system, 24
  activation, 26
  deficiency, 29, 41
Congenital infections, 62–63
Congenital rubella syndrome, 46, 62
Conidia, 8
Conjugation, 6, 102
Conjunctivitis, 44, 45
  gonococcal neonatal (ophthalmia
    neonatorum), 44, 62
Contamination, 66, 74
  soil, 100
Corneal infections, 44, 45
Coronaviruses, 114
Corynebacteria, 84
Corynebacterium diphtheriae, 34
Cotrimoxazole (trimethoprim plus
  sulphamethoxazole), 110
Coxiella burnetii, 72
Creutzfeld-Jakob disease, 14, 15, 90
Cross-infection, 94
Croup, 36
Cryptococcosis, 110
Cryptosporidiosis, 10, 76, 79, 90
Cryptosporidium parvum, 79
Culture, 30
Cyclospora spp., 90
Cyclozoonoses, 76
Cystic fibrosis, 36, 115
Cysticercosis (pork tapeworm), 64, 84,
  87, 112
Cystitis, 56
Cysts, 10
Cytokines, 24–25
Cytomegalovirus, 42, 44, 62, 72, 108
Cytoplasmic membrane, 6
Cytotoxic T cells, 26

Dapsone, 80
Defective-inferfering (DI) particles, 4
Defensins, 20, 29
Dermatophytes, 8, 48, 110
Diabetes mellitus, 52
Diagnosis, 30–31
Diarrhoea, 50
　antibiotic-associated, 50
　outbreak, case study, 78–79
　tropical infections, 84
Diethylcarbamazine (DEC), 112
Digoxin, 114
Diloxanide furoate, 112
Diphtheria, 34, 42
Disinfection, 98–99, 127
Disseminated intravascular coagulation, 46
Drug resistance, 90–91, 102
Dysentery, 50

Ebola virus, 86
Echinococcus granulosus, 42
Echocardiography, 54
Econazole nitrate, 110
Electroencephalography (EEG), 42
Elephantiasis (Bancroftian filariasis), 84, 87, 112
Emboli, 54
Enanthems, 46
Encephalitis, 42–43
　measles, 46
　meningo-encephalitis, 38
Encephalomyelitis, 42
Encephalopathies, transmissible degenerative, 14–15
Endocarditis, 104
　bacterial, 54–55, 66
　fungal, 110
Endocervicitis, 61
Endophthalmitis, 44
Endospores, 17
Endotoxins, 20, 66
Entamoeba histolytica, 79, 112
Enterobiasis, 112
Enterocolitis, 50
Epidemics, 18
Epidemiology, 18–19
Epididymo-orchitis, 38
Epiglottitis, 34
Epitopes, 29
Epstein-Barr virus, 72, 73
Ergosterol, 110
Erysipelas, 48
Erythromycin, 36, 72, 102
Escherichia coli, 38, 69, 79
　0157 strain, 90
　VTEC strains, 76
Ethambutol, 36
Ethnobotany, 114
Eukarya, 2
Eukaryotes, 2, 17
Examination, 30
Exanthems, 46
Exotoxins, 20
Eye infections, 44–45
Eyelid infections, 44
Eyeworm, 87, 112

Facial palsies, 42
Famciclovir, 108
Fansidar, 80
Fever, 69
　factitious, 88
　pyrexia of unknown origin, 88–89
　tropical infections, 84
Filaria, 12, 13
Filariasis, 84, 87, 112
Fimbriae, 6, 20
Fish-tank granuloma, 48
FitzHugh-Curtix syndrome, 52
Flagellae, 6
Flagellates, 10, 11

Flucloxacillin, 97
Fluconazole, 110
Flucytosine (5-fluorocytosine), 110
Flukes, 12, 13, 112
5-Fluorouracil, 110
Folliculitis, 48
Food
　microbiology, 100, 101
　poisoning, 50, 51, 100
Fungi, 2, 3, 8, 110
　antifungal therapy, 110–111
　dimorphic, 8, 17
　endocarditis, 110
　skin infections, 48–49
　toxins, 22
Furuncles (boils), 48

Gametocytes, 80
Ganciclovir, 108
Gangrene, 48, 64
Gas gangrene, 48
Gastroenteritis, 50, 51
　postnatal, 62
Gastrointestinal tract
　infections, 50–51
　pathogens, 20
Gene cloning, 115
Gene therapy, 115
Genetic engineering, 115
Genetically modified micro-organisms (GMOs), 115
Genital herpes, 58, 114
Genital tract infections, 58–59
Genital warts, 58
Gentamicin, 54, 56, 102, 107
Giardia lamblia, 79
Giardiasis, 84, 112
Glandular fever (infectious mononucleosis), 72, 73
Gram-stains, 6, 7, 66–67
Granuloma
　fish-tank, 48
　inguinale, 58
　swimming-pool, 48
Griseofulvin, 110
Guillain-Barré syndrome, 42

Haemagglutin, 34
Haemolysis, 17
Haemophilus spp., 107
Haemophilus ducreyi, 58
Haemophilus influenzae, 34, 36, 38, 115
　Aegyptius biogroup, 90
Haemorrhagic/petechial rashes, 46, 47
Hand-foot-and-mouth disease, 46
Handwashing, 94, 95, 97
Haptens, 29
Heart infections, 54–55
Helicobacter pylori, 22, 50, 90
Helminths, 2, 3, 12–13, 42
　antihelminthic therapy, 112, 113
　eye infections, 45
　immune response, 29
　tropical fevers, 84, 87
Helper T cells, 26
Hepatitis, viral, 52–53, 84, 108
　hepatitis B, 52, 53, 114, 115
Herbal remedies, 114
Herpes simplex virus infection
　encephalitis, 42
　genital, 58, 114
　neonatal, 62
　skin rashes, 46
Herpes zoster infection, 46, 114
Herpesviruses
　infections, 72, 73
　treatment, 108
Heterophil antibodies, 72
History, 30
HLA molecules, 26
Homoserine lactones, 114
Hookworms, 84, 87, 112

Hospital-acquired (nosocomial) infections, 66–67
　case study, 96–97
　infection control principles, 94
Host defences, 24–25
Host immunity, 20
Human immunodeficiency virus (HIV), 70–71
　drug therapy, 108, 109
Human papilloma virus (HPV), 46, 58, 108
Hyaluronidases, 20
Hyphae, 8
Hypnozoites, 80

Imaging techniques, 30
Immunisation, 116–117
Immunity, 2, 24–27
　adaptive, 24, 26–27, 74, 75, 116
　cell-mediated, 26
　evasion of, 20, 29
　herd, 116
　host, 20
　humoral, 26
　innate, 24–25, 74, 75
　short answer questions, 28–29
Immunodeficiency, 74–75
Immunogens, 29
Immunoglobulins, 26–27
　deficiencies, 29
　secretory IgA, 44, 50
Immunomodulators, 52
Immunopathology, 22–23
Immunosuppression, 74
Impetigo, 48
Incidence, 18, 94
Inclusion bodies, 22
Inclusion conjunctivitis, 44
Infection control, 2
　non-drug control, 114
　principles, 94
Infections
　acute, 18
　airway, 36
　biliary tract, 52
　bone, 64–65
　choroid, 44, 45
　chronic, 18
　congenital, 62–63
　corneal, 44, 45
　cross-infection, 94
　diagnosis, 30–31
　endemic, 18
　endogenous, 94
　epidemiology, 18–19
　eye, 44–45
　focus, 74
　gastrointestinal tract, 50–51
　genital tract, 58–59
　heart, 54–55
　hospital-acquired see Hospital-acquired infections
　host determinants of severity, 23
　hyperendemic, 18
　immunity see Immunity
　joints, 64–65
　muscle, 64
　neonatal, 62–63
　nervous system, 42–43
　new/re-emerging, 90–91
　obstetric, 62–63
　opportunist, 70–71, 74, 76
　pathogenesis, 20–21
　pathology, 22–23
　periodicity, 18
　postnatal, 62
　post-transplant, 74
　pregnancy, 62–63, 72
　prevention, 101
　resistance to, improving, 94
　skin see Skin: infections
　sources, 66, 94
　sporadic, 18

surveillance, 18, 90, 94
transmission, 18, 20, 94
tropical, 84–87
vaginal, 58, 61
virulence, 20, 23
wounds, 48, 97
Infectious agents, 2–3
Infectious mononucleosis (glandular fever),
    72, 73
Infective endocarditis see Endocarditis
Inflammation, 22, 24
Influenza, 34, 108
Interferon therapy, 46, 52, 108
Interleukins, 24
Intertrigo, 48
Intraocular infections, 44, 45
Investigations, 30
Irradiation, 98
Isoconazole, 110
Isolation rooms, 94
Isoniazid, 36
Isotypes, 26
Itraconazole, 110
Ivermectin, 112

Jaundice, 52, 114
Joints
    effusions, 64
    infections, 64–65

Kawasaki disease, 46
Keratitis, 44
Kernig's sign, 38
Ketoconazole, 110
Kinetofragminophorea, 10
Koch's postulates, 20, 21
Koplik's spots, 46

Lactobacillus spp., 24
Lactoferrin, 44
Lamivudine, 108
Lancefield grouping system, 17
Laryngotracheitis, 34
Laryngo-tracheo-bronchitis, 37
Lassa fever, 46, 76, 84, 86, 108
Latency, 4
Legionella, 74, 107
Legionella pneumophilia, 36, 90, 98, 100
Leishmaniasis, 84, 86, 112
Leprosy, 48, 84, 85
Leptospira, 6
Leukocytes, 26
Lipopolysaccharides, 20
Lipoteichoic acid, 6
Listeria, 74
Listeria monocytogenes, 38
Liver abscesses, 52, 84
Loaiasis (eyeworm), 87, 112
Lower respiratory tract infections,
    36–37
Lupus vulgaris, 48
Lymph nodes, 26, 46
Lymphadenopathies, 72
    persistent generalised, 70
Lymphocytes, 24, 26
Lymphogranuloma venereum, 58
Lysis, 4, 24
Lysogeny, 4
Lysosomes, 24
Lysozyme, 44

Macrophages, 24, 29
Macular/maculopapular rashes, 46–47
Malaria, 80–81, 84, 86, 114
    case study, 82–83
Mastigophora, 10
Mazzotti reaction, 112
Measles, 46
Mebendazole, 112
Medical microbiology, 2
Mefloquine, 80
Meglumine antimoniate, 112

Melarsoprol, 112
Meningitis, 38–39
    bacterial, 38, 39
    case study, 40–41
    tuberculous, 38
    viral, 38, 39
Meningo-encephalitis, 38
Meropenem, 107
Merozoites, 80
Metazoonoses, 76
Metronidazole, 42, 102, 112
Miconazole, 110
Microfilariae, 12, 112
Micro-organisms, 2–3
    detection, 30–31
    genetically modified (GMOs), 115
Microsporidial infections, 112
Midstream urine, 56
Minimum inhibitory concentration (MIC),
    54, 104
Molecular techniques, 30
Monocytes, 24, 26
Mosquitoes, 80
Moulds, 8
MRSA (methicillin-resistent Staphylococcus
    aureus), 94, 97, 104
Muco-ciliary escalator, 24, 36
Mucocutaneous lymph node syndrome
    (Kawasaki disease), 46
Mucosa-association lymphoid tissue
    (MALT), 26
Mumps virus
    meningitis, 38
    pancreatitis, 52
Munchausen syndrome, 88
Muscle infections, 64
Myalgia, 34
Mycelia, 8
Mycobacterium species, 6, 72, 73, 84, 98
Mycobacterium leprae, 42
Mycobacterium marinum, 48
Mycobacterium tuberculosis, 22, 48, 72, 88,
    90, 94
Mycology, 8
Mycoplasma spp., 6, 36
Mycoses, 8, 9, 110
Mycotoxins, 8, 9
Myelitis, 42
    transverse, 42, 43
Myocarditis, 38, 54, 55
Myositis, viral, 64

Natural killer cells, 24
Natural remedies, 114
Necrotizing fasciitis, 48
Neisseria gonorrhoeae, 58, 61
Neisseria meningitidis, 38, 41
Nematodes, 12, 13
Neonatal infections, 62–63
Nervous system infections, 42–43
Neuraminidase, 34
Neuritis, 42
Neurotoxins, 42
Niclosamide, 112
Nifurtimox, 112
Nitrofurantoin, 56
Nosocomial infections
    see Hospital-acquired infections
Notifiable diseases, 18, 126
Nucleoside analogues, 108
Nystatin, 110

Obstetric infections, 62–63
Onchocerciasis (river blindness), 87, 112
Oocysts, 80
Ophthalmia neonatorum, 44, 62
Opportunist infections, 70–71, 74, 76
Opsonisation, 24, 26
Orbital cellulitis, 44, 45
Osteomyelitis, 64
Otitis media, 34
Outbreaks, 18

Pancreatitis, 38, 52–53
Pandemics, 18, 90
Papillomavirus infection, 46, 58, 108
Papular/nodular rashes, 46, 47
Parasitaemia, 20
Parasites, 10
    immune response, 29
    muscle, 64
    tropical fevers, 84
    worms, 12–13, 84
    see also Helminths; Protozoa
Paratyphoid fever, 84, 85
Parenchymal infection (pneumonia), 36, 37
Paronychia, 48
Parotitis, 38
Pasteurisation, 98
Pathogenesis, 20–21
Pathogenicity islands, 20
Pathology, 22–23
PCR (polymerase chain reaction), 66
Pelvic inflammatory disease, 58
Penciclovir, 108
Penicillin, 38, 102
Penicillin V, 102
Penicillium, 110
Pentamidine, 112
Pentavalent antimony compounds, 112
Peptic ulceration, 50
Peptidogylcans, 6
Pericarditis, 54, 55
Perihepatitis, 52
Perinatal infections, 62–63
Periplasm, 6
Peritonitis, 52
Permeases, 6
Persistent generalised lymphadenopathy
    (PGL), 70
Pesticides, 115
Peyer's patches, 50
Phages, 4, 6
Phagocytic cells, 24, 26
Phagocytosis, 29
Phagolysosomes, 24
Phagosomes, 24
Pharyngitis, 34
Phosphonoformate, 108
Phyllanthrus amarus, 114
Phylogeny, 17
Phytopharmacy, 114
Piperacillin, 107
Pirodavir, 108
Pityriasis versicolor, 8
Plague, 72
    bubonic, 85
Plasma cells, 26
Plasmid DNA, 6
Plasmids, 6, 102
Plasmodium spp., 80–81, 83
Platelets, 26
Pneumocystis pneumonia, 112
Pneumonia, 36, 37
Podophyllin, 114
Poliomyelitis, 42
Polyenes, 110
Polymerase chain reaction (PCR), 66
Polyneuritis, 42
Polysaccharide capsules, 6
Porins, 6
Postnatal infections, 62
Praziquantel, 112
Pregnancy, 62–63
    systemic infections, 72
Prevalence, 18, 94
Primary lymphoid organs, 26
Prions, 3, 14, 15
Proctitis, 58
Proguanil, 80
Prokaryotes, 2, 17
Prosthetic joint infections, 64
Protozoa, 2, 3, 10–11
    antiprotozoal therapy, 112, 113
    eye infections, 45

Protozoa *(cont'd)*
  immune response, 29
  tropical fevers, 84
Pseudohyphae, 8
Pseudomembranous colitis, 50, 102
Pseudomonas, 107
Pseudomonas aeruginosa, 36, 102
Pseudopodia, 10
Psychoneuroimmunology, 114
Psychotherapy, 114
Psychrophiles, 100
Psychrotrophs, 100, 101
Public health microbiology, 100
Puerperal infections, 62
Pyelonephritis, 56
Pyknosis, 22
Pyrazinamide, 36
Pyrexia *see* Fever
Pyrimethamine, 72, 80
Pyrimidines, 110
Pyuria, sterile, 56

Q fever, 72
Quinine, 80
Quinolone, 107

Rabies, 42, 84, 86
Ramsay-Hunt syndrome, 42
Rashes, 46, 47
Reactive arthritis, 64
Reiter's syndrome, 58
Relapsing fever, 84
Renal transplant, 74
Respiratory syncytial virus (RSV), 36, 108
Respiratory tract infections, 34–35, 36–37, 97
  case study, 107
Retinal infections, 44, 45
Retinochoroiditis, 44
Retroviruses, 70
Reverse transcriptase, 70, 108
Rhinitis, 34
Rhinoviruses, 108, 114
Ribavirin, 36, 46, 52, 108
Rickettsia spp., 6, 17
Rickettsial infections, 72
Rifampicin, 36, 41
Rimantadine, 34, 108
Ringworm, 8, 48
River blindness, 87, 112
Roundworms, 12, 13, 84, 87, 112
Rubella, 46, 62

Salmonella spp., 74, 79, 90, 94, 98, 100
Saprophytes, 8
Saprozoonoses, 76
Sarcodina, 10
Sarcomastigophora, 10
Scalded skin syndrome, 48, 62
Schistosomes, 17
Schistosomiasis (bilharzia), 84, 87, 112
Schizogony, 10, 80
Schizonts, 80
Scrapie, 14
Secondary lymphoid organs, 26
Secretory IgA, 44, 50
Septic arthritis, 64
Septicaemia, 66–67
  case study, 68–69
Serology, 30–31
Sex pili, 6
Sexually transmitted diseases, 58–59
  case study, 60–61
Shigella, 79
Shock
  anaphylactic, 102
  bacteraemic, 66, 69
Short answer questions
  basic microbiology, 16–17
  immunity, 28–29
Siderophores, 20
Sinusitis, 34

Skin
  infections, 20
    bacterial, 48–49
    fungal, 48–49
    genital, 58
    mycobacterial, 48
  rashes, 46–47
  tests, 30
  tropical lesions, 84
  ulcers, 84
  viral rashes, 46–47
Sleeping sickness, 84, 86, 112
Smallpox, 46, 90, 116
Sodium artenusate, 114
Soil contamination, 100
Sore throat, 34
Specimen collection, 31
Spiramycin, 72
Spirochaetes, 6
Spleen, 26
Sporozoites, 80
Staphylococcus aureus, 20, 36, 42, 46, 48, 62, 66, 94
  methicillin-resistant (MRSA), 94, 97, 104
Sterilisation, 98–99
Stevens-Johnson syndrome, 102
Stibogluconate, 112
Streptococcus milleri, 52, 66
Streptococcus pneumoniae, 36, 38, 41, 102
Streptococcus pyogenes, 34, 35, 66, 94
Streptomyces, 110
Streptomycin, 72
Stroke, 69
Strongyloidiasis, 84, 87, 112
Styes, 44, 45
Subacute sclerosing panencephalitis, 46
Sulconazole nitrate, 110
Sulfadoxine, 80
Surveillance, 18, 90, 94
Swimming-pool granuloma, 48
Syphilis, 58, 59

T cells (T lymphocytes), 26
T helper cells, 24
Taenia solium (pork tapeworm), 64, 84, 87, 112
Tapeworms, 12, 13, 64, 84, 87, 112
Taxonomy, 17
Teichoic acid, 6
Terbinafine, 110
Tetanus, 42
Tetracyclines, 72, 102
Thiabendazole, 112
Thrombocytopaenia, 46
Thymus, 26
Thyroiditis, 38
Tick typhus, 84
Tinea (ringworm), 8, 48
Tinidazole, 112
Tonsillitis, 34
TORCH, 62
Toxins, 20, 21, 22
Toxocara spp., 42
Toxoplasma gondii, 72
Toxoplasmosis, 10, 62
Tracheitis, 34
Trachoma, 44
Transduction, 6, 102
Transformation, 6
Transmissible degenerative
  encephalopathies (TDE), 14–15
Transplants
  post-transplant infections, 74
  xenotransplantation, 90, 115
Transposons (jumping genes), 102
Trematodes (flukes), 12, 13, 112
Treponema, 6
Treponema pallidum, 58
Trichinella spiralis, 64
Trichomonas vaginalis, 61
Trichomoniasis, 10, 112
Trichuriasis (whipworm), 84, 87, 112
Trimethoprim, 56

Tropheryma whippelii, 90
Tropical infections, 84–87
Trypanosoma spp., 42, 112
Trypanosoma cruzi, 64
Trypanosomiasis
  African, 84, 86, 112
  American, 64, 84, 86
Tuberculin test, 72, 88
Tuberculosis, 36, 37, 72, 84, 85
  meningitis, 38
  urinary tract infections, 56
Typhoid fever, 84, 85
Typhus, endemic, 85

Ulcers
  peptic, 50
  skin, 84
  tropical, 85
Upper respiratory tract infections, 34–35
Urethral syndrome, 56
Urethritis, 58, 61
Urinary catheters, 56
  specimens (CSU), 69
Urinary tract infections, 56–57, 69, 97

Vaccines, 116–117
Vaginal infections, 58, 61
Vaginosis, 58
Valaciclovir, 108
Vancomycin, 54, 97, 102
Vancomycin-resistant enterococci (VRE), 104, 107
Varicella-zoster virus, 42, 74, 108
Vectors, 10
Vegetations, 54
Vesicular/pustular rashes, 46, 47
Vincent's organisms, 84
Viral haemorrhagic fevers, 46, 47
Viral load, 70
Virions, 4, 14
Viroids, 14
Virulence, 20, 23
Viruses, 2, 3, 4–5
  AIDS, 70
  antiviral therapy, 108
  cerebrospinal fluid, 42
  classification, 4
  evasion of immune response, 29
  families, 5
  hepatitis *see* Hepatitis
  meningitis, 38, 39
  new, 90
  replication, 4
  skin rashes, 46–47
  structure/morphology, 4
  terminology, 17
  tissue damage, 22
  tropical fevers, 84
Vitamin C, 114

Warts, 46
  genital, 58
Water microbiology, 100
Whipworms, 84, 87, 112
White cell count, 30
Whooping cough, 36, 116
Window period, 70
Worms, parasitic, 12–13, 84
Wound abscesses, 48
Wound infections, 48, 97

Xenotransplantation, 90, 115

Yeasts, 8, 110
Yellow fever, 86
Yersinia pestis, 72

Ziehl-Neelsen stain, 6
Zinc, 114
Zooanthropozoonoses, 76
Zoonoses, 10, 42, 72, 76–77
  case study, 78–79